Hatha Yoga Asanas

Pocket Guide for Personal Practice

Hatha Yoga Asanas

POCKET GUIDE FOR PERSONAL PRACTICE

Daniel DiTuro ■ Ingrid Yang

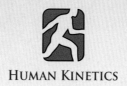

HUMAN KINETICS

Library of Congress Cataloging-in-Publication Data

DiTuro, Daniel.
  Hatha yoga asanas : pocket guide for personal practice / Daniel DiTuro,
Ingrid Yang.
    p. cm.
  ISBN-13: 978-1-4504-1485-2 (soft cover)
  ISBN-10: 1-4504-1485-0 (soft cover)
  1. Hatha yoga. I. Yang, Ingrid, 1979- II. Title.
  RA781.7.D58 2012
  613.7'046--dc23
                            2011041296

ISBN-10: 1-4504-1485-0 (print)
ISBN-13: 978-1-4504-1485-2 (print)

The web addresses cited in this text were current as of November 2011, unless otherwise noted.

Developmental Editor: Laura E. Podeschi; **Assistant Editor:** Tyler Wolpert; **Copyeditor:** Jan Feeney; **Cover Designer:** Keith Blomberg; **Photographer (cover and interior):** Daniel DiTuro; **Photo Production Manager:** Jason Allen; **Printer:** United Graphics

We thank the owners of Prana Yoga Center in La Jolla, California, and Yoga is Youthfulness in Mountain View, California, for assistance in providing the locations for the photo shoots for this book.

Human Kinetics books are available at special discounts for bulk purchase. Special editions or book excerpts can also be created to specification. For details, contact the Special Sales Manager at Human Kinetics.

Printed in the United States of America   10 9 8 7 6 5 4 3 2 1

The paper in this book is certified under a sustainable forestry program.

Human Kinetics
Website: www.HumanKinetics.com

United States: Human Kinetics
P.O. Box 5076
Champaign, IL 61825-5076
800-747-4457
e-mail: humank@hkusa.com

Canada: Human Kinetics
475 Devonshire Road Unit 100
Windsor, ON N8Y 2L5
800-465-7301 (in Canada only)
e-mail: info@hkcanada.com

Europe: Human Kinetics
107 Bradford Road
Stanningley
Leeds LS28 6AT, United Kingdom
+44 (0) 113 255 5665
e-mail: hk@hkeurope.com

Australia: Human Kinetics
57A Price Avenue
Lower Mitcham, South Australia 5062
08 8372 0999
e-mail: info@hkaustralia.com

New Zealand: Human Kinetics
P.O. Box 80
Torrens Park, South Australia 5062
0800 222 062
e-mail: info@hknewzealand.com

E5537

Contents

THE ASANAS   1

SUN SALUTATION   159

Acknowledgments

This book would not have been possible without the enthusiastic dedication of dozens of yoga teachers and students whom I've had the great pleasure of working with over the years. They volunteered their time and talent as an extension of their love of yoga. Each photo session allowed me the opportunity to expand my appreciation of the diversity yoga offers to men and women of all ages. I am extremely thankful to have worked with so many gifted people on this project.

This undertaking would not have been possible without the support and encouragement of my parents, Donato and Rachele DiTuro. They immigrated from a rural part of southern Italy to the United States for new opportunities. Their dedication and vision ensured that their children would have a better life. My parents allowed me to pursue my love of cooking, science, and the arts. They were excellent teachers with little formal education. They never attended a cooking or science class nor the opera or symphony, but they excelled at cooking, were enthralled by science, and enjoyed all music, from classical to pop. I cannot thank them enough for their love and the many sacrifices they made in pursuing a better life.

The photographs in this book were shot in Arizona and California. For allowing me to use their yoga studios for the California photo shoots, I thank Sabina Hentz, co-owner of Yoga Is Youthfulness in Mountain View, and Gerhard Gessner and Alexandra Oehmigen-Gessner, owners of Prana Yoga Center in La Jolla.

Special thanks to Cheri Gross for coordinating the Mountain View photo shoot. Cheri devoted many hours recruiting excellent yoga teachers to model for the book, assigning the poses for each model, and arranging for the use of Yoga Is Youthfulness.

I met my coauthor, Ingrid Yang, at the La Jolla photo shoot. Her sincere enthusiasm for the project was evident from the very beginning. She assisted with setup and teardown and modeled for a fast-paced photo session scheduled between yoga classes. I learned from Ingrid how many asanas have evolved over the years, placing more emphasis on the physical abilities of the majority rather than the extreme flexibility of a minority. It was a pleasure working with Ingrid on this book.

More than 20 yoga teachers and students modeled for this book over a period of seven years. They endured less-than-ideal conditions modeling many of the asanas without complaint. Their professionalism was amazing. Each photo session taught me a new pose or variation of a pose. Each photo shoot, like each model, was unique. I learned so much in the process. The models' experience ranged from gentle to vigorous ashtanga vinyasa yoga.

The models appearing in this book are Ingrid Yang, Pamela Scott, Elizabeth Ormon, Beth Perry, Cheri Gross, Carlos Mendez, Louis Jackson, Beata Skrzypacz, Zahra Mojdeh Zahiraleslamzadeh, Liza DiGaetano, Gerhard Gessner, Jamie Pinkum, Kristi Nelson, Justina Kerth, Robert Birks, and Leslie Thompson. You are all awesome, and I thank each of you for your time and the opportunity to work with you on this project.

Finally, my gratitude to Jason Muzinic and Human Kinetics for the opportunity to make this book available to all yogis and yoginis.

Daniel DiTuro

The adage "It takes a village to raise a child" applies to writing a book. I owe thanks to every person who has come into my life to challenge, support, embrace, or inspire me. Among the many people to whom I owe thanks, the first is my cousin Sharon, who supported, encouraged, and believed in me when it seemed that no one else did. Her faith in my ability to succeed and fulfill my dreams has never wavered and, consequently, has passed onto me. I owe to Sharon my belief in positive self-fulfilling prophecies, tenacity, and unquestioning love.

Special thanks to my teachers Sarah Trelease, Cyndi Lee, David Life, Sharon Gannon, and Dharma Mittra. Your wisdom and guidance will continue to resonate with me throughout my life. To the community of Blue Point Yoga Center in Durham, North Carolina, thank you for allowing me to be your founder, teacher, and fearless leader for many years. To the community at Prana Yoga Center in La Jolla, California, and Alex Gessner, thank you for welcoming me with open arms and offering me the opportunities, support, and enthusiasm to teach new and innovative programs. I am especially indebted to Gerhard Gessner, a true yogi in his own right, for guiding me on this path by his example.

Thanks to Lululemon Athletica for providing some of the models' outfits and specifically to the teams at Lululemon Athletica in La Jolla and Bucktown, Chicago, for being my biggest fans and supporters.

I owe particular thanks to Daniel DiTuro for spearheading this project. Your deft organizational skills, superb photography skills, and great attitude have made you a true joy to work with on this project. I could not have asked for a better partner in writing this book.

To Beth Perry for being a superb yoga model and writing consultant.

To Seiji Ike-Glenn (www.neblite.com), my amazing website programmer, who presents my content to the world in a logical, streamlined, and aesthetically beautiful platform. You are a technical and artistic genius.

To Gabe Feenberg (Old Man Hands) for working with me to create beautiful music that will inspire yogis and enhance the practice of yoga everywhere. Gabe, you are a rare, brilliant musical talent, and I am truly honored to have shared a microphone with you.

To my parents for giving me all the opportunities, moral guidance, and patience that a daughter could ask for. Thank you for instilling in me the values that have made me the person I am today. I owe you everything.

And finally, to every yoga student I have been so fortunate to teach, it is a privilege to be your teacher, and in turn, you have been my teachers.

Ingrid Yang

Introduction

The English translation of the Sanskrit word *yoga* is "union." It means that, despite the physical, spiritual, and emotional boundaries people erect among themselves in modern life, humans are, on the most basic level, one and the same. Our goal for this book is to embody this concept of common humanity by exploring the many manifestations of hatha yoga asanas as physical expressions of this connectedness.

The numerous documented physical and mental benefits of hatha yoga have played a large part in our interest in yoga in the West. The benefits of hatha yoga include reduced blood pressure, relief from stress and anxiety, improved flexibility, and decreased muscle and joint pain. While the people of India have long known the healing power of hatha yoga, this practice and its benefits are relatively new to most people in the West. As Western medicine has embraced the mental and physical benefits of hatha yoga, it has become more prominent in everyday life. However, brief references to yoga in the media and the various marketing departments promoting paraphernalia to capitalize on the practice have done little to define it for would-be practitioners.

Hatha yoga is the yoga of asanas (postures). While it is only one of eight limbs of yoga codified by Patanjali, it is what most people associate with yoga when it is mentioned in everyday vernacular. It seems that you cannot visit a coffee shop or attend a dinner party without overhearing or being engaged in a conversation about yoga. Even a person who has never practiced yoga will recognize the lotus pose. The irony is that the lotus asana was developed to enhance one's ability to meditate for long periods and connect to a deep sense of spirituality and calm being. Interestingly, calm meditation is the opposite of what many seek when they practice hatha yoga.

Most of the asanas associated with hatha yoga were developed less than 100 years ago and have evolved into hundreds of variations. This evolution has occurred so that you can adapt hatha yoga into modern life and the realities of your present existence. No two people are exactly alike. Modifying postures to your ability is what sets hatha yoga apart from many other physical activities. Not everyone can play football or basketball, run a fast mile, or climb mountains, but almost everyone can enjoy and benefit from some form of hatha yoga. There are no limits in terms of age, height, or weight. We selected diverse models, both male and female, to demonstrate the universal appeal of hatha yoga and to emphasize that the power of its practice extends beyond the boundaries of physicality.

Here, we come back to the concept that underlies the practice of yoga and our perspective in writing this book: We are one. Despite differing shapes and constitutions, we as humans share the link of humanity and a collective yearning to discover the truth within ourselves. That truth can be uncovered through the practice of hatha yoga, because how you relate to your inner self can be revealed through outer expression. As you explore the intricate world of hatha yoga asanas, you should never lose sight of the larger picture.

For newcomers to hatha yoga, learning the asana names can be as confusing as learning a new language. It is difficult enough to learn the English names of the postures while practicing in a yoga class. Once an instructor begins using Sanskrit names, it is easy for new students to become confused. Sanskrit is an ancient foreign language and many of the asana names sound alike to the untrained ear. They all end in *asana*, which, although loosely translated to "posture," really means "seat." In that regard, recalling that you are always entering a position of repose with each asana is a useful practice whether you are an overwhelmed novice or a more seasoned yogi.

This book is a quick guide to over 150 classic hatha yoga asanas, which are taught in a variety of yoga classes and every training course for yoga teachers. The asanas range from gentle yoga for beginners to more advanced physical forms of yoga. Most styles of hatha yoga teach two or three dozen of the asanas in this book, but that should not prevent you from exploring new poses to expand and enhance your practice. You may discover after studying one style of yoga that you are ready to advance to, or try, another style. One of the greatest benefits of yoga is the ability to modify your practice to your needs, whether physical, mental, or both.

If you practice yoga, are a yoga teacher, or are considering becoming a yoga teacher, this book will serve as a comprehensive resource for learning the yoga asanas along with their English names, Sanskrit names, and levels of difficulty. The difficulty ratings in this book are based on the following criteria:

- ▶ Flexibility
- ▶ Strength
- ▶ Balance

The rating of difficulty is a relative guide: The easiest asanas are rated 1 and the most difficult are rated 10. Of course, what is easy for one person may be extremely difficult for someone else. That is to be expected since every person's physical abilities vary depending on age, physical condition, health conditions, and numerous other factors. You might execute a perfect tree pose one day but be unable to repeat the same pose the next.

This is the dharma (teaching) that is accepted as part of yoga practice. As with any physical activity, improvement comes with practice. Range of motion, mental alertness, strength, stamina, and focus will all improve with regular and dedicated practice. These are some of the reasons medical doctors are recommending hatha yoga to their patients.

The asanas in this book are listed in alphabetical order by their traditionally accepted English names translated from Sanskrit. Most asanas named after deities, sages, or heroic figures are listed by their English names. For example, galavasana is listed as sage galava, not flying crow pose. Exceptions are virabhadrasana, which is commonly referred to as warrior rather than hero virabhadra. The Sanskrit name is also included for each asana.

The popularity of hatha yoga has resulted in dozens of variations of a given pose. One teacher's extended triangle pose is another's extended side stretch. This can be confusing if you are accustomed to practicing one style of hatha yoga and then are introduced to another style. For most people, variations are a necessity. Limited flexibility and your specific body structure can prevent you from executing some of the poses in this book. We encourage the use of props and variations to modify any pose to your ability. Being flexible enough to sit in lotus or wrap your legs behind your head is not indicative of good yoga practice. Instead, a sense of calm, contentment, and focus in each pose is the true foundation of yoga practice.

The models in this book are yoga practitioners and teachers representing various levels and styles of hatha yoga, including ashtanga, vinyasa, and Iyengar. These styles of yoga trace their lineage to Tirumalai Krishnamacharya, a Brahmin born in the 19th century in a South Indian village. He developed ashtanga vinyasa yoga while teaching at the Sanskrit College in Mysore, India. Thanks to the devotion of his student K. Pattabi Jois and Jois' students, ashtanga yoga is one of the most popular styles of physical hatha yoga in the West. Another student of Krishnamacharya, B.K.S. Iyengar, is one of the most influential teachers of hatha yoga. Not only is his style one of the most popular styles of hatha yoga in the West, but many of Iyengar's students also have gone on to promote yoga and even develop their own styles of yoga. Iyengar is known for precisely aligned postures and for promoting the healing benefits of yoga. While most yoga teachers specialize in one or two forms of yoga, Krishnamacharya modified yoga postures for the infirm, for pregnant women, and for children. The creator of the physically and mentally challenging ashtanga vinyasa yoga also designed the much gentler viniyoga style, which is taught by his son T.K.V. Desikachar.

The instructions in this book are based on principles developed by B.K.S. Iyengar. They are simplified instructions for achieving each asana. Our best suggestion is to take your time, listen to your body, and breathe, regardless of where you are in your yoga practice.

Vinyasa yoga is a series of postures linked into a continuous routine. Surya namaskara, the sun salutation, is perhaps the most well known of these routines. There are as many variations of the sun salutation as there are asanas. The sun salutation in this book is one of many variations ideal for home practice. Each takes only a few minutes and can be done anywhere at any time.

Perhaps most important, yoga is simply a practice. It is not a science, a strict regimen, or a religion. There will be no finish line or complete product. It is simply the daily practice of awakening to each moment and discovering what emerges. Yoga teaches you to meet each moment as it arises without judgment, just as it is. Although we sought to depict asanas in this book as they are practiced aspirationally, our message is that yoga is truly for everyone. Yoga provides a path to greater awareness and unity of mind, body, and spirit. May this book guide you throughout your journey.

The Asanas

Bharadvaja's Twist

Bharadvajasana

Difficulty Level 4

Start Position Hero (p. 74)

1 Keep right leg in hero and extend left leg forward.

2 Bend left knee, turning left foot into right hip.

3 Twist to left, holding left foot with left hand behind back, and place right hand on outer left thigh.

4 Gaze over left shoulder. Repeat on other side.

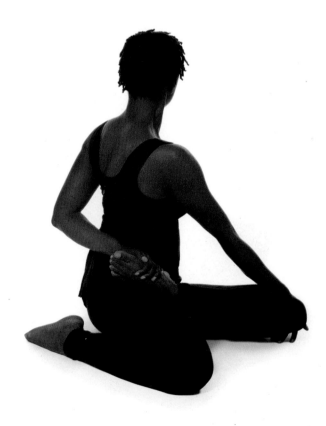

Big-Toe Hold, Both

Ubhaya Padangusthasana

Difficulty Level   5

Start Position   Staff (p. 139)

1 Bend knees and curl first two fingers around big toes.

2 Extend legs straight.

3 Look toward feet and balance on sit bones.

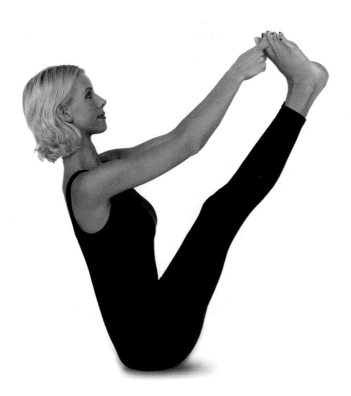

Big-Toe Hold, Reclining

Supta Padangusthasana

Difficulty Level 5

Start Position **Reclining on back**

1 Bend right knee and curl first two fingers around big toe.

2 Straighten leg upward and toward head. Repeat on other side.

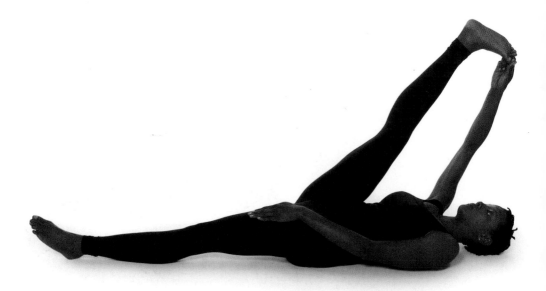

Big-Toe Hold, Reclining Side

Supta Parsva Padangusthasana

Difficulty Level 4

Start Position Reclining on back

1 Bend right knee and curl first two fingers around big toe.

2 Straighten leg upward and toward head.

3 Rotate right arm and leg to right side. Repeat on other side.

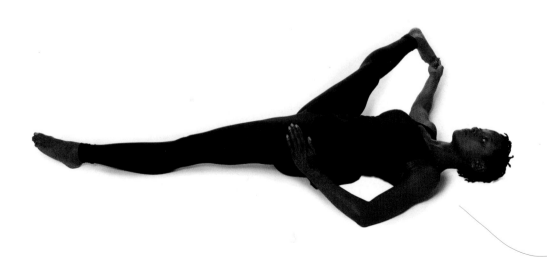

Boat, Full

Paripurna Navasana

Difficulty Level 5

Start Position Boat, half (p. 7)

1 Extend legs straight, maintaining extended spine.

2 Lengthen fingers beyond knees.

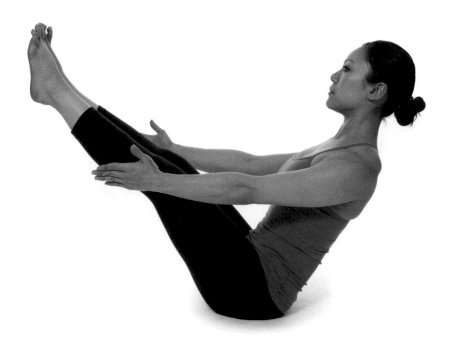

Boat, Half

Ardha Navasana

Difficulty Level   4

Start Position   Staff (p. 139)

1 Bend knees, lean back, and balance on sit bones.

2 Lift feet so that shins are parallel to floor.

3 Reach fingers beyond knees.

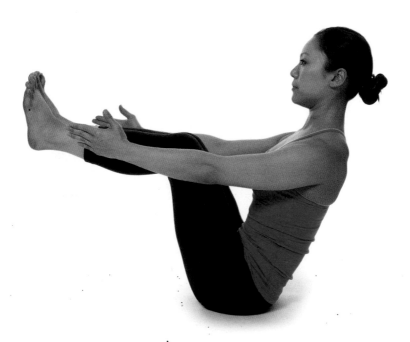

Bound Angle

Baddha Konasana

Difficulty Level 2

Start Position Staff (p. 139)

1 Bend knees toward chest, and draw feet close to body.

2 Hold feet with hands and open knees out to each side.

3 Sit tall and relax belly and hips.

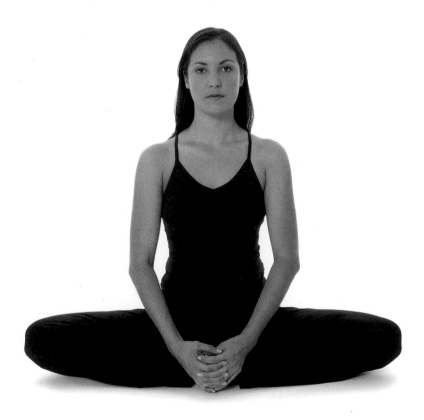

Bound Angle, Extended

Utthita Baddha Konasana

Difficulty Level 2

Start Position Bound Angle (p. 8)

1 Hold feet and fold forward with extended spine.

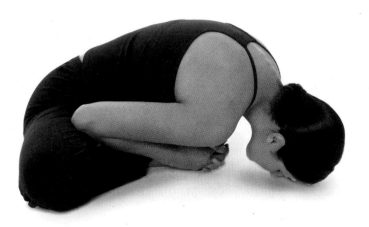

Bound Angle, Reclining

Supta Baddha Konasana

Difficulty Level   3

Start Position   Bound angle (p. 8)

1 Walk elbows behind body until reclining.

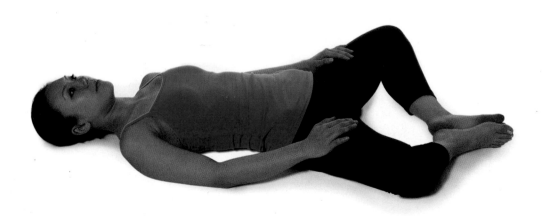

Bow

Dhanurasana

Difficulty Level 5

Start Position Lying on belly

1 Bend knees and clasp hands onto feet or ankles.

2 Kick feet back, lifting thighs and chest away from floor.

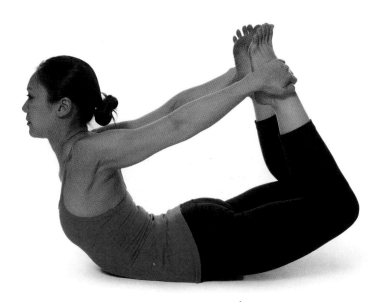

Bow, Big Toe

Padangustha Dhanurasana

Difficulty Level 9

Start Position Lying on belly

1 Place hands on floor under shoulders and straighten arms into a backbend.

2 Bend both knees and stretch one arm overhead to catch both feet.

3 Lift other hand back to clasp foot and hold one foot in each hand.

4 Bend elbows and arch head back, touching head to feet.

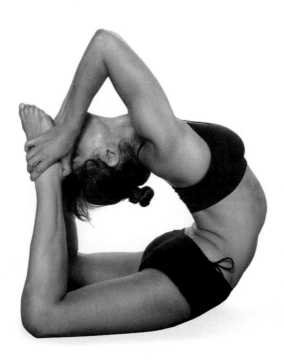

Bow, Side

Parsva Dhanurasana

Difficulty Level   6

Start Position   Bow (p. 11)

1 Maintaining hold of ankles, roll onto left side of body.

2 Roll back into bow and repeat on right side.

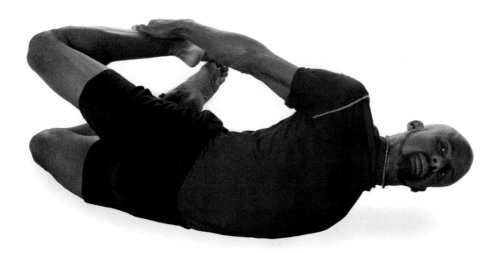

Bridge

Setu Bandha Sarvangasana

Difficulty Level   4

Start Position   **Reclining on back**

1 Bend knees, stepping feet on floor, with arms alongside body.

2 Press into feet, lifting hips; walk arms and shoulders toward each other.

3 Place hands on lower back, or keep arms on floor and interlace fingers.

4 Walk feet directly below knees and lift chest toward chin.

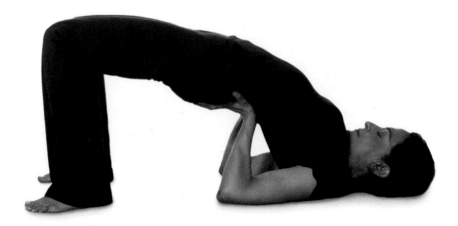

Camel

Ustrasana

Difficulty Level   6

Start Position   Kneeling (p. 81)

1 Raise hips to stand on knees and shins.

2 Lean back to reach for heels with hands, keeping hips above knees.

3 Relax head back or keep chin tucked into chest.

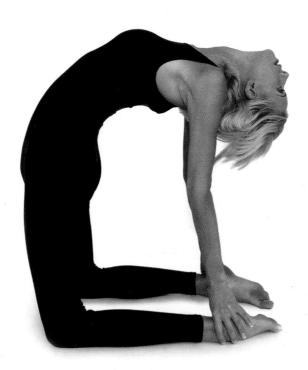

Cat

Marjaryasana

Difficulty Level 2

Start Position Child's (p. 18)

1 Come forward to align hips over knees and shoulders over wrists in neutral spine.

2 Round spine on exhale, pulling belly in and chin to chest.

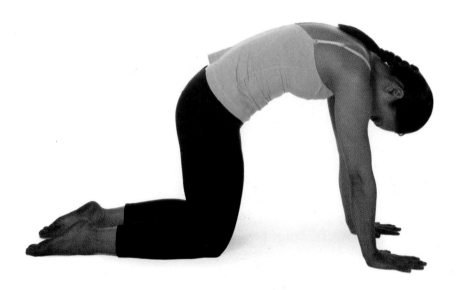

Chair

Utkatasana

Difficulty Level 3

Start Position Mountain, standing (p. 96)

1 Bend knees, sitting back in hips.

2 Lift arms alongside head.

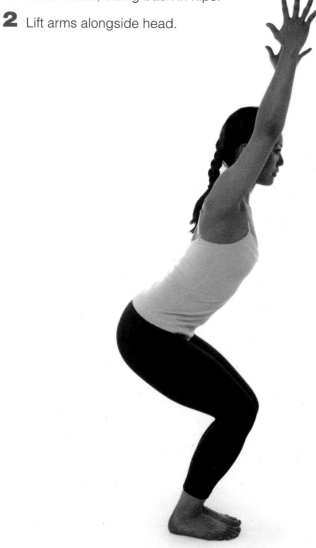

Child's

Balasana

Difficulty Level 1

Start Position Kneeling (p. 81)

1 Rest buttocks toward heels and lean over thighs.

2 Touch forehead to floor.

3 Extend arms alongside body.

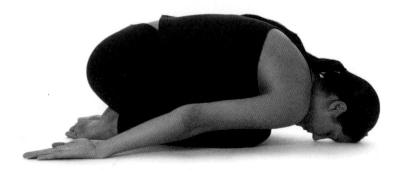

Child's, Extended

Utthita Balasana

Difficulty Level 1

Start Position Child's (p. 18)

1 Extend arms forward.

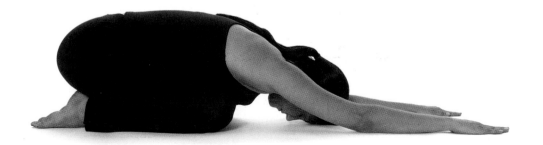

Cobra

Bhujangasana

Difficulty Level   4

Start Position   **Lying on belly**

1 Place hands under shoulders.

2 Straighten arms slowly, lifting chest; gaze forward.

3 Keep tops of thighs and feet on floor.

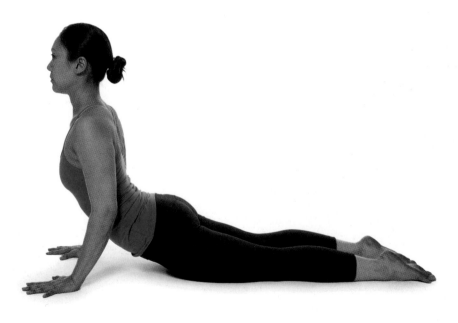

Cobra, Half

Ardha Bhujangasana

Difficulty Level 3

Start Position **Lying on belly**

1 Place hands alongside ribs.

2 Slide chest forward and slightly up, keeping belly on floor.

3 Extend through crown of head and keep shoulders drawn back.

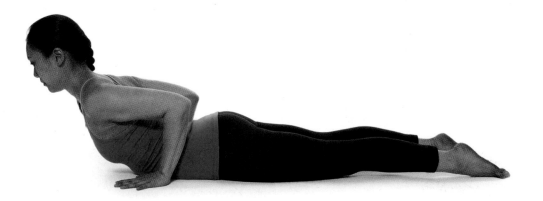

Cock

Kukkutasana

Difficulty Level 8

Start Position Lotus, seated (p. 90)

1 Thread arms under knees with legs remaining in lotus.

2 Lean forward and place hands on floor.

3 Straighten arms to balance buttocks and legs off floor.

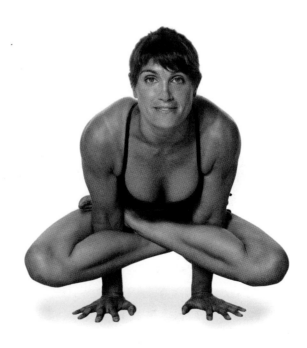

Cock, Side

Parsva Kukkutasana

Difficulty Level 9

Start Position Lotus, seated (p. 90)

1 Twist to right side and place hands on floor.

2 Press strongly into hands to lift body, and hook left thigh onto right triceps.

3 Lean forward and straighten arms and balance. Repeat on other side.

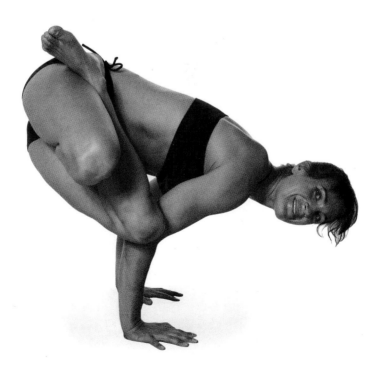

Cock, Upward

Urdhva Kukkutasana

Difficulty Level 9

Start Position Lotus, seated (p. 90)

1 Bend knees up into chest, remaining in lotus, and walk hands in front of body.

2 Bend arms and shift shins onto triceps.

3 Lean forward and straighten arms.

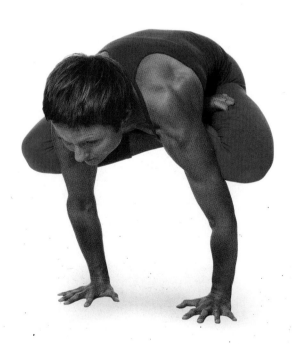

Cord

Pasasana

Difficulty Level 5

Start Position Garland I (p. 60)

1 Draw knees and feet together and twist to left.

2 Hook right shoulder outside of left thigh and extend left arm behind back.

3 Clasp right hand around left wrist. Repeat on other side.

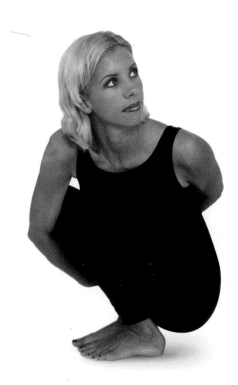

Corpse

Savasana

Difficulty Level 1

Start Position **Reclining on back**

1 Close eyes.

2 Let feet fall apart and palms face sky.

3 Relax and let go of breath.

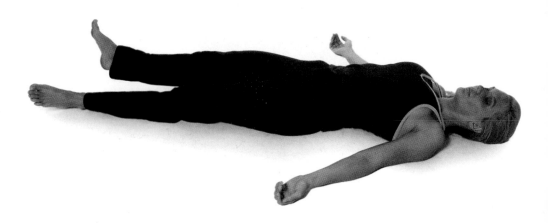

Couch

Paryankasana

Difficulty Level   4

Start Position   Hero (p. 74)

1 Walk elbows back and lie on upper back.

2 Hold opposite elbows.

3 Arch back and place crown of head on floor with chest lifted.

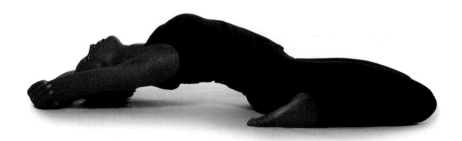

Cow

Bitilasana

Difficulty Level 2

Start Position Child's (p. 18)

1 Come forward and align hips over knees and shoulders over wrists in neutral spine.

2 Drop belly toward floor with heart lifted and pelvis tilted back.

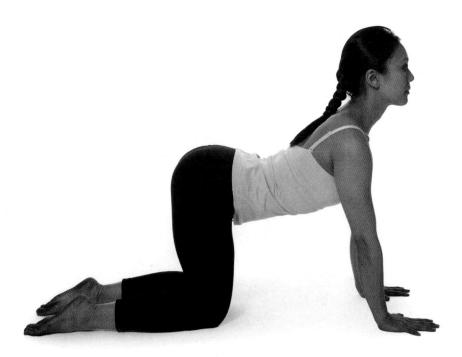

Cow Face

Gomukhasana

Difficulty Level 4

Start Position Kneeling (p. 81)

1 Cross right knee over left knee and sit in between heels.

2 Extend left arm up, bending elbow.

3 Extend right arm back, clasping hands behind back. Repeat on other side.

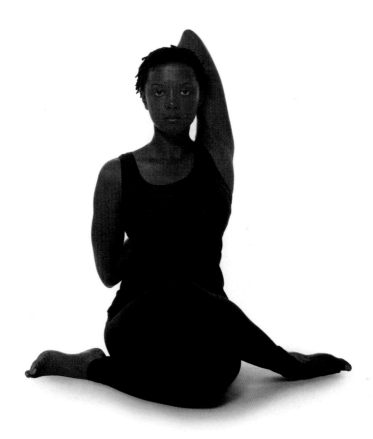

Cradle

Eka Padasana

Difficulty Level 2

Start Position **Easy sitting (p. 41)**

1 Lift right shin parallel to chest.

2 Wrap crooks of elbows around foot and knee.

3 Maintain long spine to hug shin to chest. Repeat on other side.

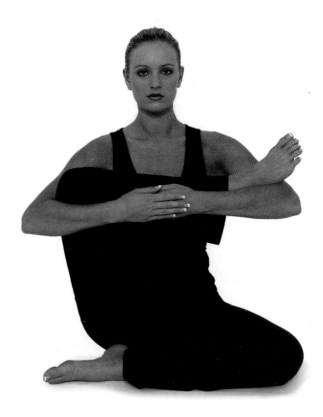

Crescent Lunge

Anjaneyasana

Difficulty Level 3

Start Position Downward-facing dog (p. 39)

1 Step left foot between hands and relax right knee to floor.

2 Lift arms above head, backbending and lifting chest. Repeat on other side.

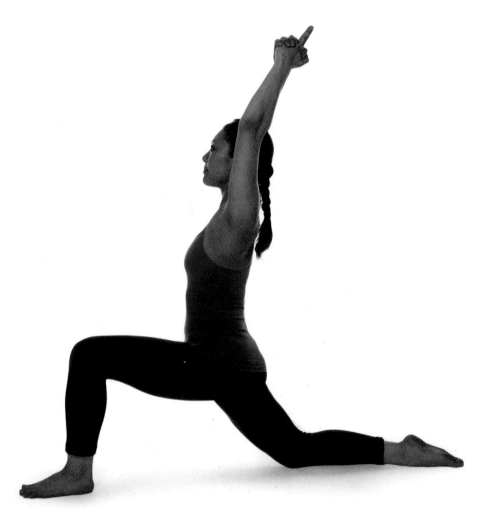

Crescent Moon

Ashta Chandrasana

Difficulty Level 3

Start Position Mountain, standing (p. 96)

1 Lift arms alongside head.

2 Lean to left, keeping even weight on both feet. Repeat on other side.

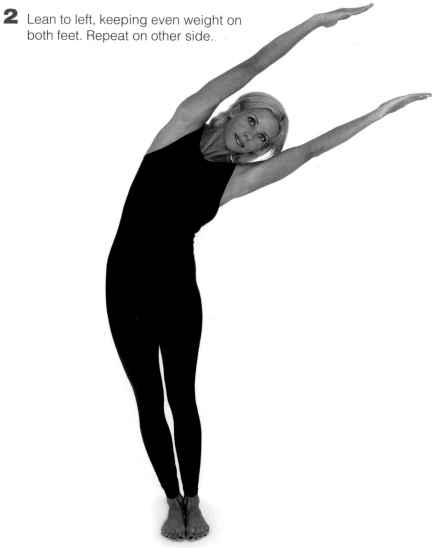

Crow

Bakasana

Difficulty Level   5

Start Position   Garland I (p. 60)

1 Walk hands in front of feet and lift onto tiptoes.

2 Hug knees into upper arms and lean forward to balance on hands.

3 Straighten arms.

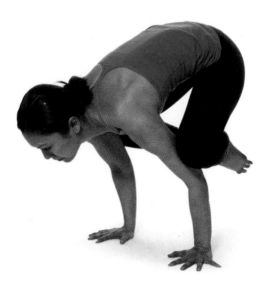

Crow, One Leg

Eka Pada Bakasana

Difficulty Level 7

Start Position Crow (p. 33)

1 Extend left leg back in the air. Repeat on other side.

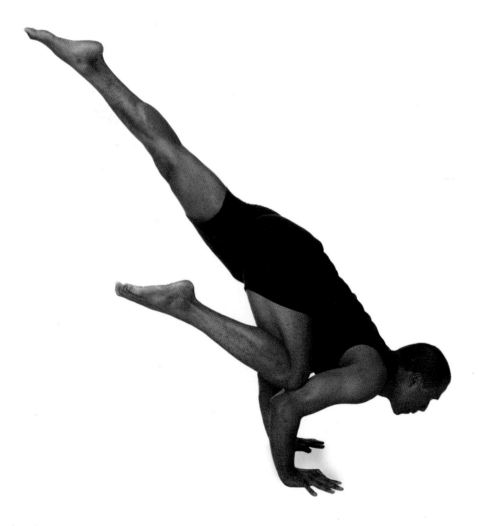

Crow, Side

Parsva Bakasana

Difficulty Level 6

Start Position Chair (p. 17)

1 Hook left triceps to outer right thigh, squatting down until hands reach floor.

2 Shift weight forward, lifting feet off floor. Repeat on other side.

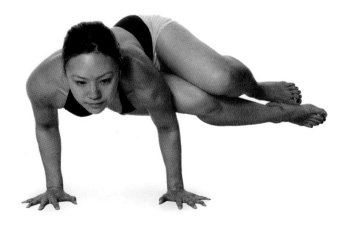

Dancer I

Natarajasana I

Difficulty Level 5

Start Position Mountain, standing (p. 96)

1 Bend right leg and catch right foot or ankle in right hand.

2 Kick leg back, extending chest forward and backbending.

3 Reach left arm forward. Repeat on other side.

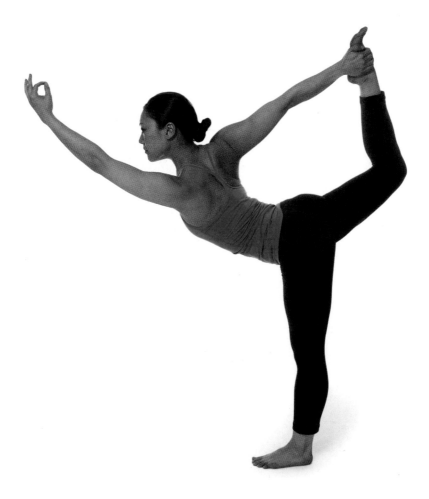

Dancer II

Natarajasana II

Difficulty Level 8

Start Position Mountain, standing (p. 96)

1 Bend left leg; with internally rotated arm, catch left inner foot with left hand.

2 Lift left leg with left hand overhead, rotating left shoulder to turn left elbow upward.

3 Reach right arm overhead to also catch left foot.

4 Continue backbending, extending chest forward. Repeat on other side.

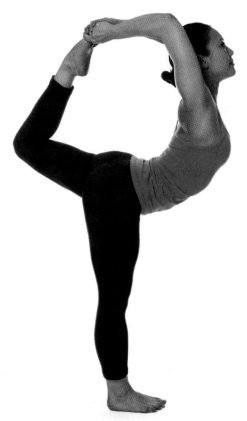

Dancer III

Natarajasana III

Difficulty Level 7

Start Position Dancer II (p. 37)

1 Extend left arm forward while keeping hold of left foot with right hand. Repeat on other side.

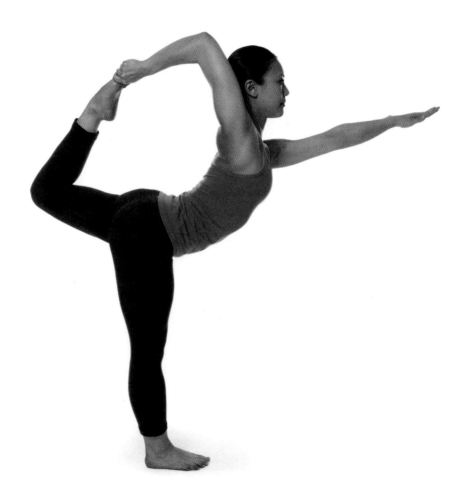

Downward-Facing Dog

Adho Mukha Svanasana

Difficulty Level 3

Start Position Plank (p. 106)

1 Press hips upward and back.

2 Relax chest toward feet with ears alongside upper arms.

3 Extend heels toward floor, stretching backs of legs.

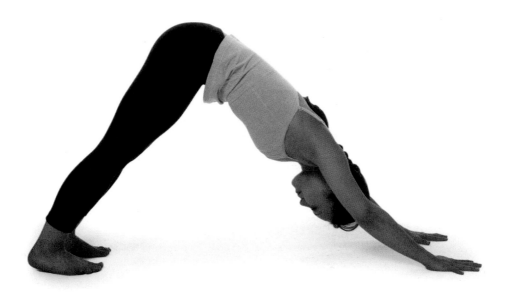

Ear Pressure

Karnapidasana

Difficulty Level   5

Start Position   Plow (p. 109)

1 Bend knees alongside ears.

2 Extend arms on floor and interlace fingers.

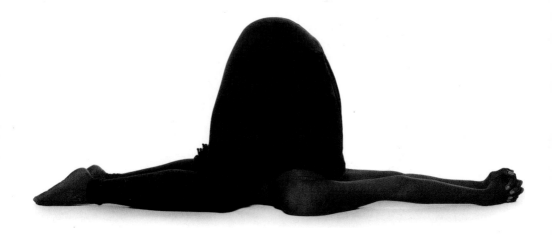

Easy Sitting

Sukhasana

Difficulty Level 1

Start Position Staff (p. 139)

1 Bend right foot toward body, rotating right hip so right knee rests on floor.

2 Bend left knee, aligning left foot in front of right or crossing over right ankle.

3 Repeat on other side.

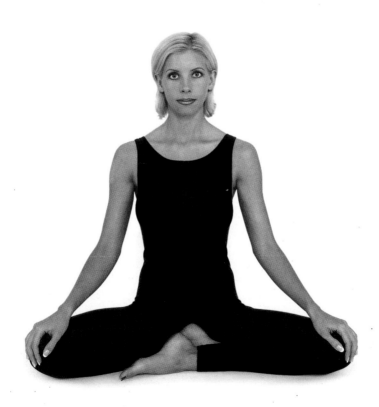

Eight Angle

Astavakrasana

Difficulty Level   7

Start Position   Easy sitting (p. 41)

1 Hook right shoulder under right knee and extend left leg forward on floor.

2 Place hands on floor on either side of left thigh.

3 Press into hands, lifting buttocks off floor and hooking left ankle over right ankle.

4 Bend elbows, moving chest forward, and extend legs to right side. Repeat on other side.

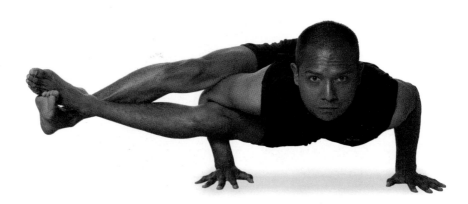

Elephant's Trunk

Eka Hasta Bhujasana

Difficulty Level 6

Start Position Easy sitting (p. 41)

1 Hook left shoulder under left knee and extend right leg.

2 Place hands on floor on either side of right thigh.

3 Press into hands and lift entire body off floor, keeping right leg parallel to floor. Repeat on other side.

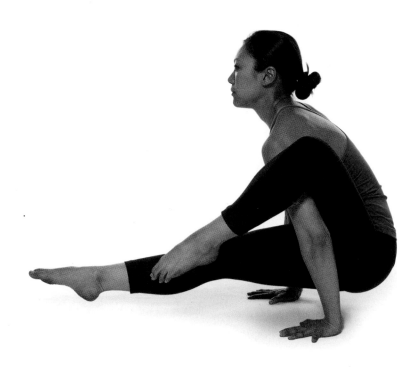

Embryo in Womb

Garbha Pindasana

Difficulty Level 7

Start Position Lotus, seated (p. 90)

1 Thread arms under calves, remaining in lotus.

2 Balance on upper buttocks, lifting legs into chest, and hold ears with hands.

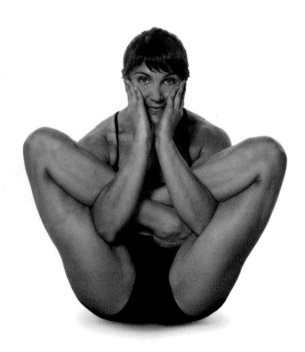

Firefly

Tittibhasana

Difficulty Level 7

Start Position Garland I (p. 60)

1 Lift hips and walk hands behind feet, creating a shelf with triceps.

2 Sit on triceps and extend legs out to sides.

3 Straighten arms.

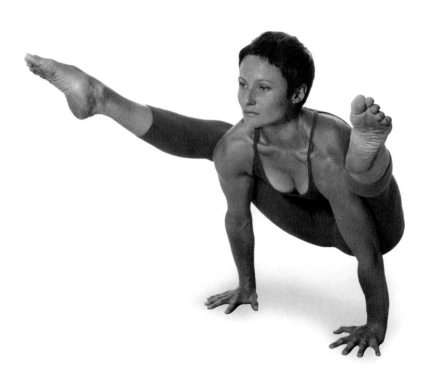

Fish

Matsyasana

Difficulty Level 3

Start Position **Reclining on back**

1 Bend elbows to floor and slide hands under buttocks.

2 Lift chest by pressing elbows into floor, and relax crown of head to floor.

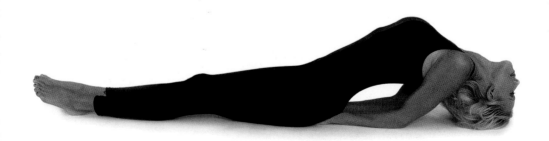

Fish, Lotus

Padma Matsyasana

Difficulty Level 5

Start Position **Reclining on back**

1 Cross legs into lotus.

2 Bend elbows on floor and slide hands under buttocks.

3 Lift chest by pressing elbows into floor, and relax crown of head to floor.

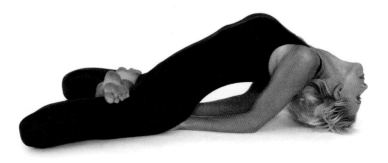

Foot Behind Head

Eka Pada Sirsasana

Difficulty Level   8

Start Position   Staff (p. 139)

1 Hold outer left foot with right hand and duck head under left shin.

2 Extend right leg forward and lean back into left leg.

3 Place hands to prayer at heart. Repeat on other side.

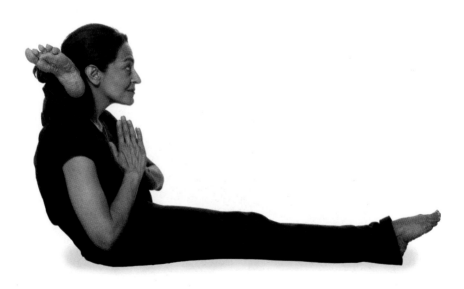

Forward Bend, Seated

Paschimottanasana

Difficulty Level   4

Start Position   Staff (p. 139)

1 Fold forward, hinging at hips.

2 Hold on to feet or opposite wrist and relax head to legs.

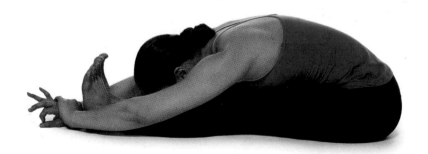

Forward Bend, Seated Half Bound Lotus

Ardha Baddha Padma Padmottanasana

Difficulty Level 4

Start Position Staff (p. 139)

1 Bend right leg into lotus.

2 Reach right hand behind back to hold right foot.

3 Fold over extended left leg, holding left foot with left hand. Repeat on other side.

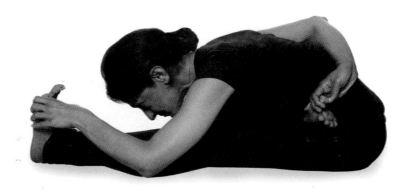

Forward Bend, Seated Head to Knee

Janu Sirsasana

Difficulty Level 4

Start Position Staff (p. 139)

1 Bend left knee and place left foot into inner right thigh.

2 Fold forward over right leg, holding foot or opposite wrist. Repeat on other side.

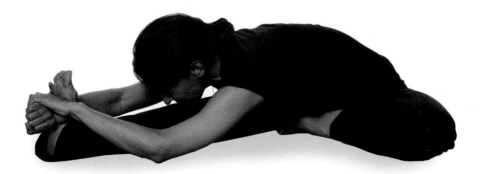

Forward Bend, Seated Wide Angle

Upavistha Konasana

Difficulty Level   4

Start Position   Staff (p. 139)

1 Extend legs to sides, externally rotating thighs.

2 Catch hold of feet or big toes and fold chest forward with extended spine.

3 Maintan external rotation in the hips and grounding in thighs.

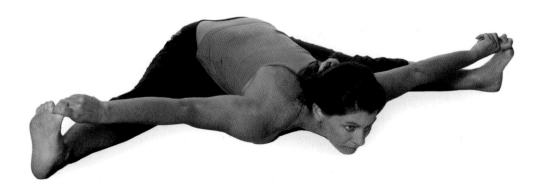

Forward Bend, Standing Big Toe

Padangusthasana

Difficulty Level   4

Start Position   Mountain, standing (p. 96)

1 Fold forward from hips, tilting sit bones up.

2 Curl first two fingers of hands around big toes, relaxing crown of head to floor.

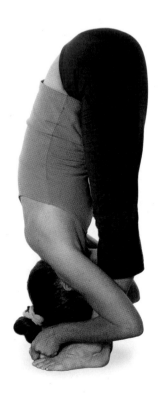

Forward Bend, Standing Hands to Feet

Padahastasana

Difficulty Level 5

Start Position Mountain, standing (p. 96)

1 Fold forward from hips, tilting sit bones up.

2 Walk hands under feet, palms facing up.

3 Relax crown of head to floor.

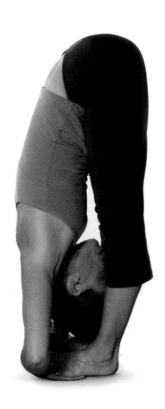

Forward Bend I, Standing

Uttanasana I

Difficulty Level 4

Start Position Mountain, standing (p. 96)

1 Fold forward, hinging at hips and tilting sit bones up.

2 Place hands on floor next to feet.

3 Relax head to floor.

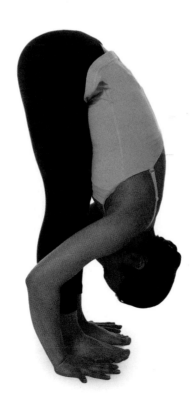

Forward Bend I, Standing Wide Leg

Prasarita Padottanasana I

Difficulty Level 4

Start Position Mountain, standing (p. 96)

1 Step feet into a wide-leg stance with parallel feet.

2 Fold forward from hips, tilting sit bones up.

3 Keep fingers parallel with toes and relax crown of head to floor.

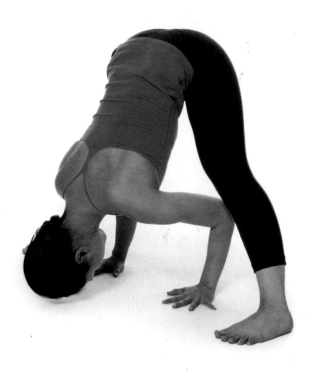

Forward Bend II, Standing

Uttanasana II

Difficulty Level 4

Start Position Mountain, standing (p. 96)

1 Fold forward, hinging at hips and tilting sit bones up.

2 Hold on to backs of legs to draw head closer to legs.

3 Relax head to floor.

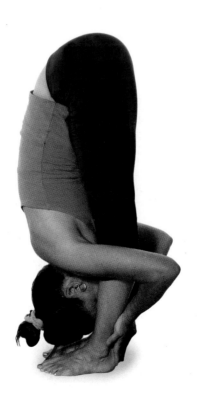

Forward Bend II, Standing Wide Leg

Prasarita Padottanasana II

Difficulty Level 4

Start Position Mountain, standing (p. 96)

1 Step feet into a wide-leg stance with parallel feet.

2 Fold forward from hips, tilting sit bones up.

3 Curl first two fingers around big toes, relaxing crown of head to floor.

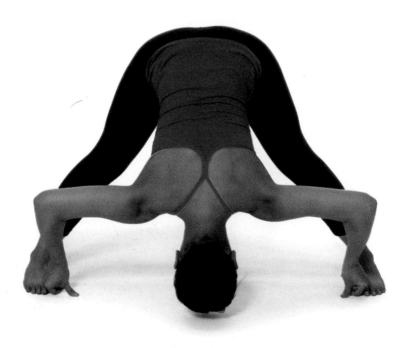

Frog

Bhekasana

Difficulty Level 6

Start Position **Lying on belly**

1 Bend one leg at a time next to hips and catch toes with hands.

2 Press chest forward and upward.

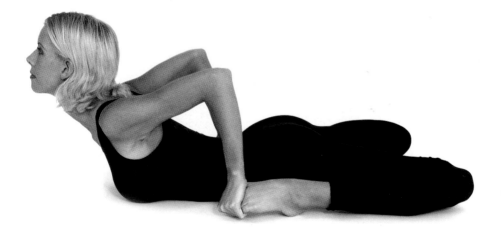

Garland I

Malasana I

Difficulty Level 4

Start Position Mountain, standing (p. 96)

1 Squat down in between thighs.

2 Brings hands to prayer position at heart.

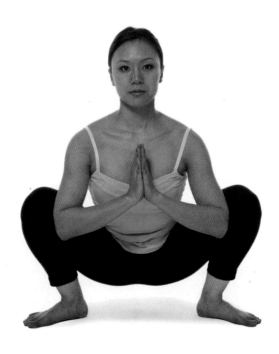

Garland II

Malasana II

Difficulty Level   4

Start Position   Garland I (p. 60)

1 Hold backs of heels with hands.

2 Extend forward, relaxing head to floor.

3 Hold on to heels or extend arms forward.

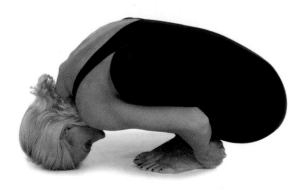

Gate

Parighasana

Difficulty Level 3

Start Position Kneeling (p. 81)

1 Kneel in an upright position, extending left leg to side.

2 Slide left hand to shin or foot and extend right arm overhead to left. Repeat on other side.

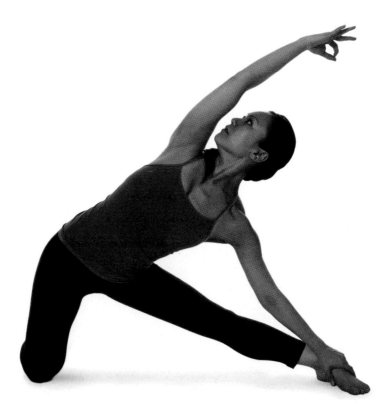

God of War

Skandasana

Difficulty Level 7

Start Position Staff (p. 139)

1 Bend left leg behind head.

2 Fold forward over extended right leg, catching hold of left wrist with right hand. Repeat on other side.

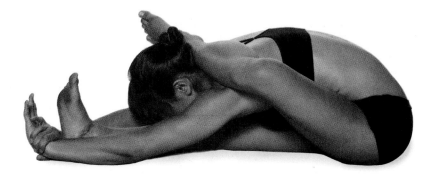

Half Moon

Ardha Chandrasana

Difficulty Level   5

Start Position   Warrior II (p. 152)

1 Place right fingers on floor forward of right foot.

2 Extend left leg back and left arm up.

3 Straighten both legs and gaze upward. Repeat on other side.

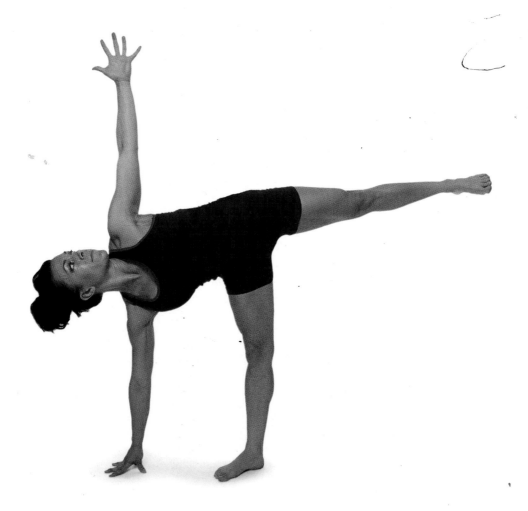

Hand to Big Toe, Extended

Urdhva Padangusthasana

Difficulty Level   6

Start Position   Mountain, standing (p. 96)

1 Bend right knee up to chest, and hold onto foot with hands or curl first two fingers around big toe.

2 Straighten right leg forward and up. Repeat on other side.

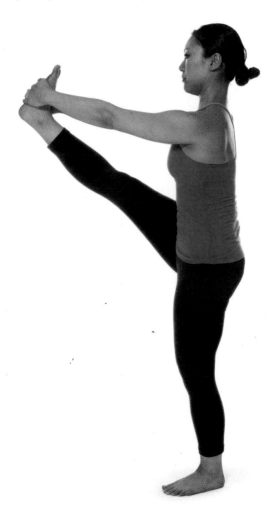

Hand to Big Toe, Extended Side

Utthita Parsva Hasta Padangusthasana

Difficulty Level 6

Start Position Mountain, standing (p. 96)

1 Bend left knee into chest, curling first two fingers around big toe.

2 Straighten left leg forward and rotate to left side. Repeat on other side.

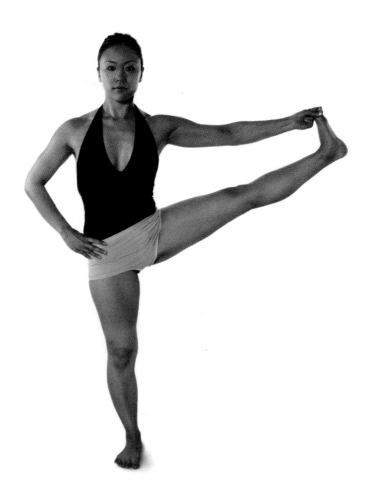

Handstand

Adho Mukha Vrksasana

Difficulty Level	7
Start Position	Downward-facing dog (p. 39)

1 Walk feet forward a few steps and extend one leg back and upward.

2 Keep hips square and bend bottom leg to hop both legs up into balance. Repeat on other side.

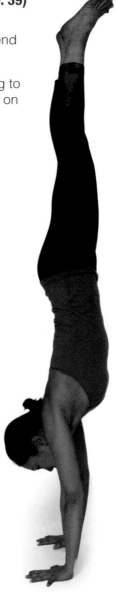

Happy Baby

Ananda Balasana

Difficulty Level   2

Start Position   Reclining on back

1 Hold outsides of feet with hands.

2 Bend knees into armpits.

3 Extend sacrum to floor.

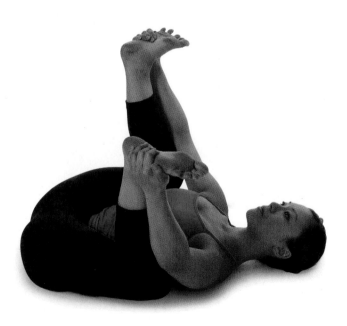

Head to Knee, Revolved

Parivrtta Janu Sirsasana

Difficulty Level 3

Start Position Forward bend, seated head to knee (p. 51)

1 Extend left leg toward left side.

2 Turn torso toward right bent knee and stretch sideways along extended left leg.

3 Hold inner arch of left foot with left hand.

4 Reach right arm overhead for left toes. Repeat on other side.

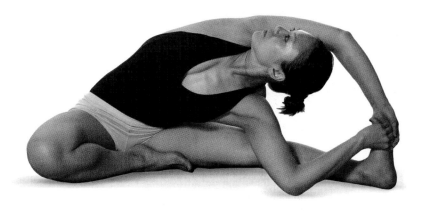

Headstand, Eagle

Garuda Salamba Sirsasana

Difficulty Level 6

Start Position Headstand, supported (p. 72)

1 Separate legs and cross left leg over right.

2 Hook left foot behind right ankle. Repeat on other side.

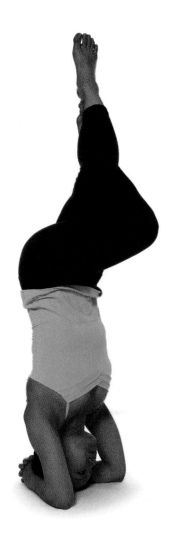

Headstand, One-Leg Revolved

Parivrttaikapada Sirsasana

Difficulty Level 6

Start Position Headstand, supported (p. 72)

1 Separate legs and rotate legs clockwise.

2 Reverse and rotate legs counterclockwise.

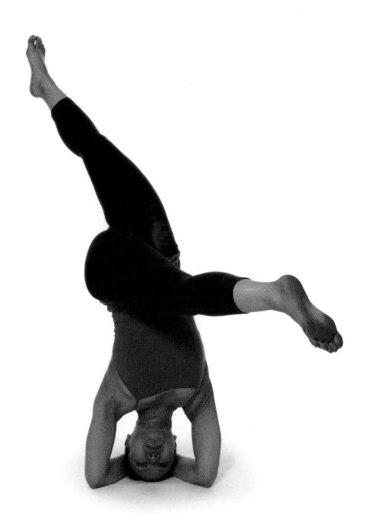

Headstand, Supported

Salamba Sirsasana

Difficulty Level   6

Start Position   Downward-facing dog (p. 39)

1 Bend elbows to floor and interlace fingers; relax crown of head between wrists.

2 Walk feet toward head until hips are over shoulders.

3 Lift one leg at a time or both together until feet extend straight up.

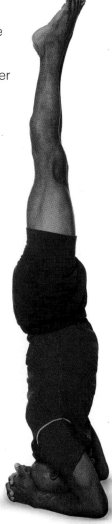

Heavenly Spirits

Valakhilyasana

Difficulty Level 7

Start Position Pigeon, one-leg king of (p. 105)

1 Catch hold of back leg with both hands.

2 Extend leg toward floor, backbending. Repeat on other side.

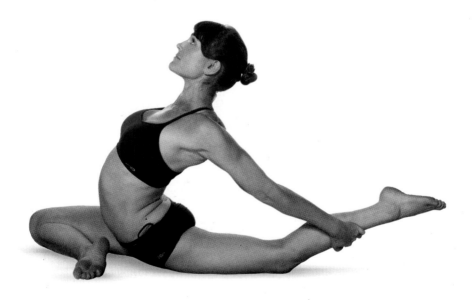

Hero

Virasana

Difficulty Level   4

Start Position   Kneeling (p. 81)

1 Separate feet and sit hips to floor between feet.

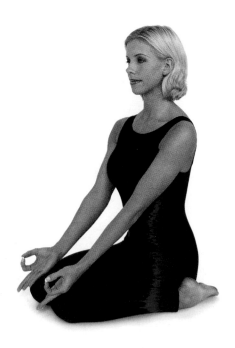

Hero, Reclining

Supta Virasana

Difficulty Level   4

Start Position   Hero (p. 74)

1 Walk elbows back until reclining.

2 Extend arms overhead.

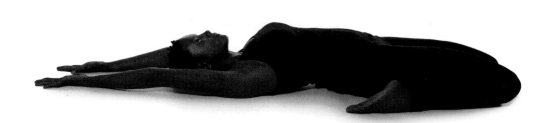

Heron

Krounchasana

Difficulty Level 5

Start Position Hero (p. 74)

1 Extend right leg and wrap both hands around right foot.

2 Lift right leg toward head. Repeat on other side.

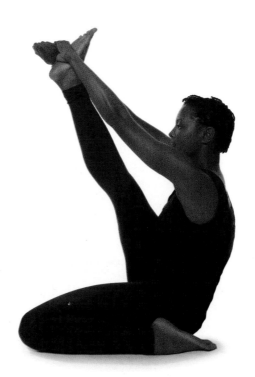

Horse Face

Vatayanasana

Difficulty Level 7

Start Position Kneeling (p. 81)

1 Rotate left leg into lotus.

2 Push up to balance on right foot and left knee.

3 Thread left arm under right and connect palms. Repeat on other side.

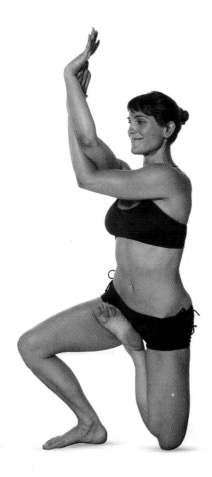

Inclined Plane

Purvottanasana

Difficulty Level 4

Start Position Staff (p. 139)

1 Walk hands back, fingers pointing toward sit bones.

2 With hands under shoulders, press hips upward and toes to floor.

3 Hang head back or keep chin tucked to chest.

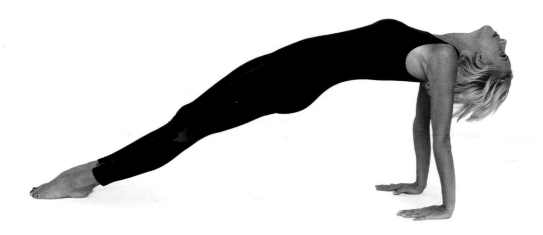

Intense Three-Limb Stretch

Trianga Mukhaikapada Paschimottanasana

Difficulty Level   6

Start Position   Hero (p. 74)

1 Extend right leg forward.

2 Fold forward over right leg and bind hands. Repeat on other side.

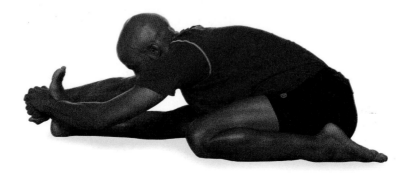

Inverted Staff, One Leg

Eka Pada Viparita Dandasana

Difficulty Level   7

Start Position   Wheel, full (p. 154)

1 Walk elbows to floor and interlace fingers.

2 Walk feet forward to straighten legs.

3 Extend one leg up. Repeat on other side.

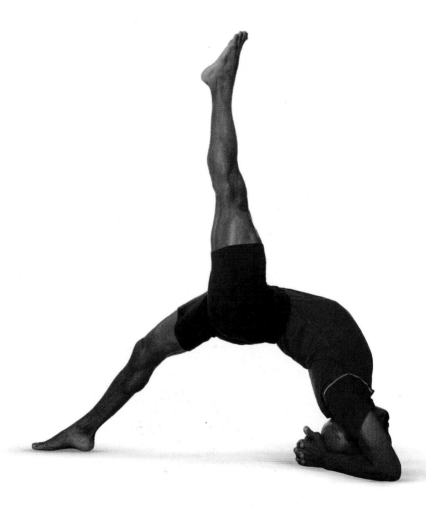

Kneeling

Vajrasana

Difficulty Level 1

Start Position Kneeling

1 While kneeling, sit on heels.

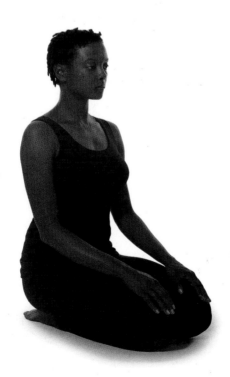

Leg Lift, Extended

Urdhva Prasarita Padasana

Difficulty Level 2

Start Position Reclining on back

1 Extend arms overhead.

2 Lift legs until feet are above hips.

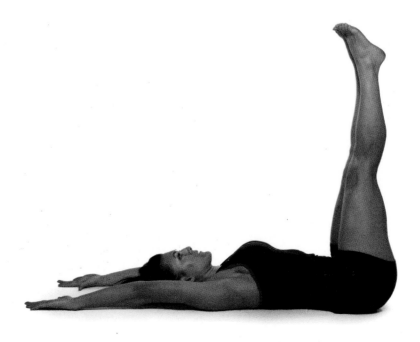

Leg Lift, Side Reclining

Anantasana

Difficulty Level 4

Start Position Reclining on left side

1 Bend left arm and place hand under head.

2 Curl first two right fingers around right big toe and extend right leg up. Repeat on other side.

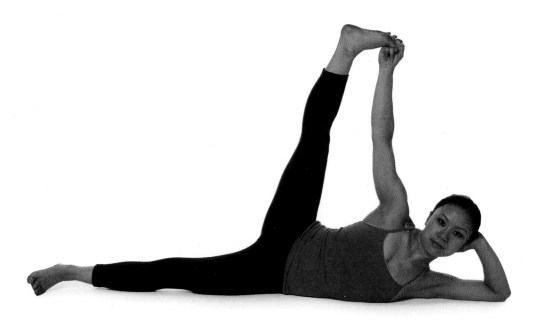

Lion

Simhasana

Difficulty Level 2

Start Position Kneeling (p. 81)

1 Cross ankles and sit on heels.

2 Hold knees with hands and exhale through mouth, sticking out tongue.

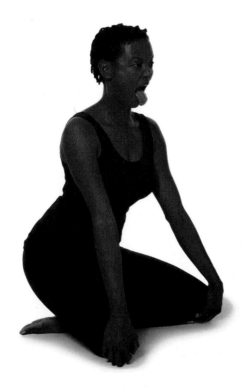

Locust

Salabhasana

Difficulty Level 3

Start Position Cobra, half (p. 21)

1 Extend arms alongside body.

2 Lift thighs and chest off floor and extend toes back.

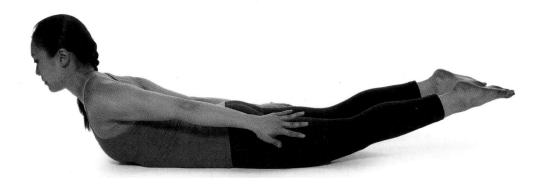

Looking Within

Sanmukhi Mudra

Difficulty Level   3

Start Position   Lotus, seated (p. 90)

1 Cover eyes with fingers and lift elbows so they are level with shoulders.

2 Place thumbs over ear holes.

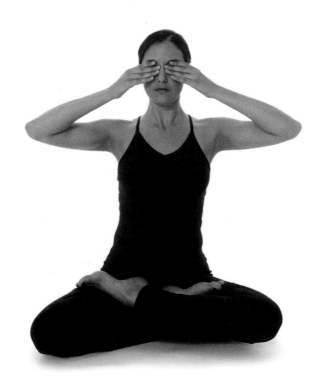

Lord of the Fishes, Half

Ardha Matsyendrasana

Difficulty Level   3

Start Position   Easy sitting (p. 41)

1 Step right foot in front of bent left knee.

2 Hook left elbow outside of right thigh, keeping sit bones on floor.

3 Twist, look over left shoulder, and clasp right wrist in left hand. Repeat on other side.

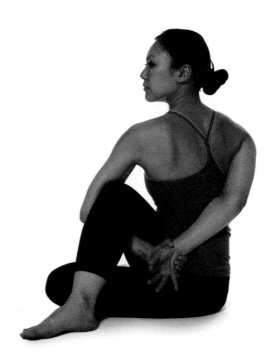

Lotus, Handstand

Padma Adho Mukha Vrksasana

Difficulty Level 8

Start Position Handstand (p. 67)

1 Bend legs into lotus, staying in hand balance, and lower knees to hip height.

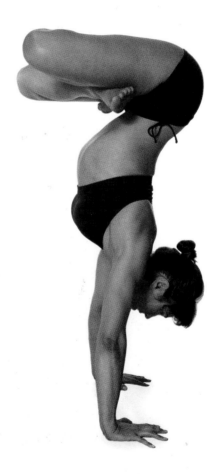

Lotus, Headstand

Padma Sirsasana

Difficulty Level 7

Start Position Headstand, supported (p. 72)

1 Bend legs into lotus, staying in head balance, and lower knees to hip height.

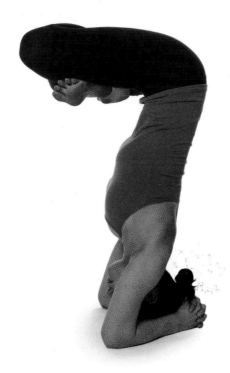

Lotus, Seated

Padmasana

Difficulty Level 3

Start Position Staff (p. 139)

1 Bend right knee, rotating from hip, and place right foot into left hip crease.

2 Rotate left hip to bend left leg over right, placing left foot into right hip crease.

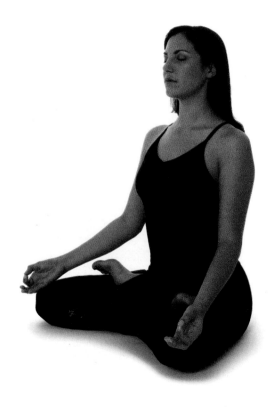

Lotus, Seated Bound

Baddha Padmasana

Difficulty Level   5

Start Position   Lotus, seated (p. 90)

1 Cross arms behind back and reach for opposite big toes.

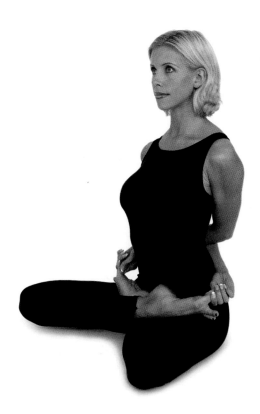

Lotus, Seated Half

Ardha Padmasana

Difficulty Level 2

Start Position Easy sitting (p. 41)

1 Bend left knee, rotating from hip, and place left foot into right hip crease.

2 Repeat on other side.

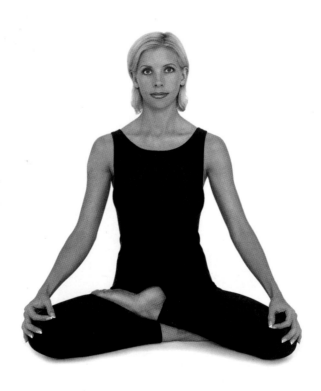

Lotus, Standing Half Bound

Ardha Baddha Padmasana

Difficulty Level 5

Start Position Mountain, standing (p. 96)

1 Bend left knee, rotating from hip, and place left foot into right hip crease.

2 Extend left arm behind waist, catching hold of left foot. Repeat on other side.

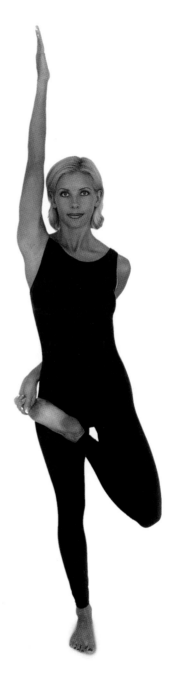

Lotus, Standing Half Bound Forward Bend

Ardha Baddha Padmottanasana

Difficulty Level   4

Start Position   Mountain, standing (p. 96)

1 Bend left knee, rotating from hip, and place left foot into right hip crease.

2 Extend left arm behind waist, catching hold of left foot.

3 Fold forward, resting right hand on floor. Repeat on other side.

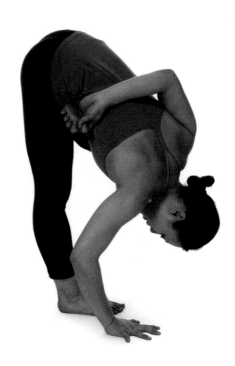

Mountain, Seated Lotus

Padma Parvatasana

Difficulty Level 3

Start Position Lotus, seated (p. 90)

1 Interlace fingers and extend palms to sky.

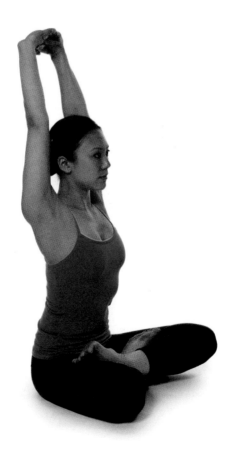

Mountain, Standing

Tadasana

Difficulty Level	1
Start Position	Standing

1 Stand with feet hip-width apart and relax arms alongside body.

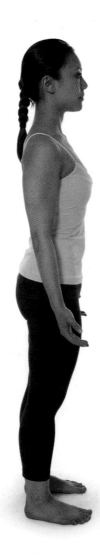

Noble Sealing

Maha Mudra

Difficulty Level	2

Start Position	Staff (p. 139)

1 Extend left leg, bending right foot into left thigh.

2 Clasp fingers around big toe and lift belly toward spine and perineum up and in. Repeat on other side.

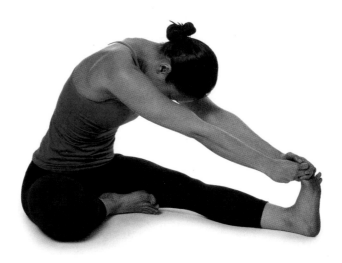

Partridge

Kapinjalasana

Difficulty Level 8

Start Position Plank, side (p. 107)

1 Bend top leg and reach top arm overhead to clasp toes.

2 Kick foot back to backbend. Repeat on other side.

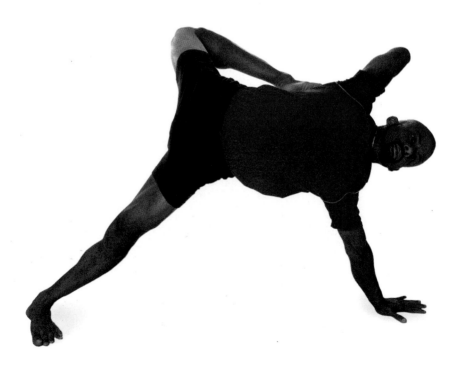

Peacock

Mayurasana

Difficulty Level 8

Start Position Kneeling (p. 81)

1 Bend elbows into belly.

2 Lean forward onto hands, pointing fingers back.

3 Extend legs back, parallel to floor.

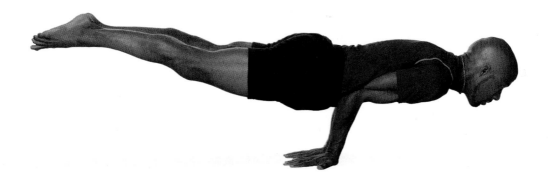

Peacock, Lotus

Padma Mayurasana

Difficulty Level 8

Start Position Lotus, seated (p. 90)

1 Bend elbows into belly, coming to stand on top of knees.

2 Lean forward onto hands, fingers pointing back.

3 Extend knees back, parallel to floor.

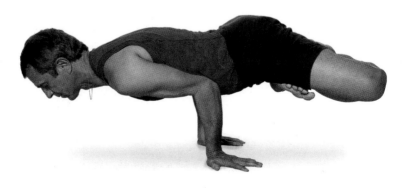

Peacock Feathers (Forearm Stand)

Pincha Mayurasana

Difficulty Level 7

Start Position Downward-facing dog (p. 39)

1 Bend elbows to floor, keeping forearms parallel.

2 Extend right leg up with hips square, and bend left knee to hop into balance. Repeat on other side.

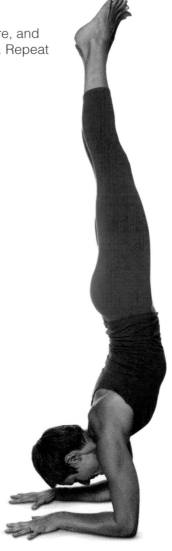

Pendant

Lolasana

Difficulty Level 8

Start Position Kneeling (p. 81)

1 Lift hips and cross ankles.

2 Place hands on floor on both sides of body.

3 Lift legs off floor and balance knees up toward chest.

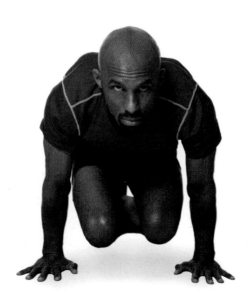

Pigeon

Kapotasana

Difficulty Level   6

Start Position   Camel (p. 15)

1 Stand on knees and lean back.

2 Extend arms overhead until hands reach floor.

3 Shift hips to sky and walk hands to feet until forearms and head rest on floor.

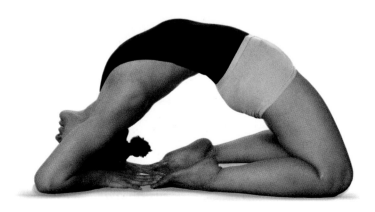

Pigeon, King of

Rajakapotasana

Difficulty Level   10

Start Position   Lying on belly

1 Place hands on floor under shoulders to backbend and bend knees to head.

2 Clasp one knee at a time to hold both knees, and arch head back toward feet.

3 With hands, pull feet and head together.

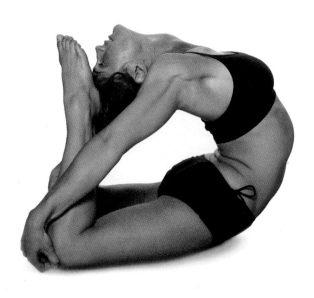

Pigeon, One-Leg King of

Eka Pada Rajakapotasana

Difficulty Level 7

Start Position Downward-facing dog (p. 39)

1 Bend right knee and place it behind right wrist with left leg extended back.

2 Bend left knee and reach overhead with one hand, then both, for left foot.

3 Arch back, reaching crown of head toward left foot. Repeat on other side.

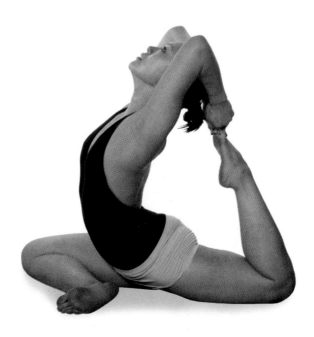

Plank

Phalankasana

Difficulty Level 2

Start Position **Lying on belly**

1 Position hands under shoulders and forehead against floor.

2 Press into hands and straighten arms, lengthening heels backward and crown of head forward.

3 Keep belly lifted and hips in line with body.

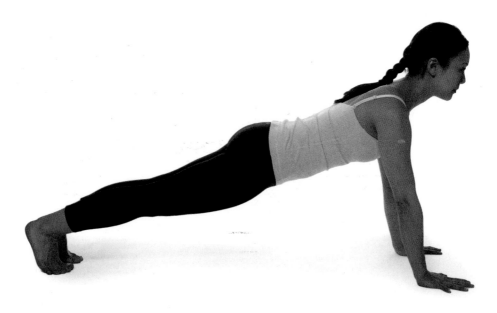

Plank, Side

Vasisthasana

Difficulty Level 6

Start Position Plank (p. 106)

1 Rotate onto left hand and stack right foot over left.

2 Extend right hand upward. Repeat on other side.

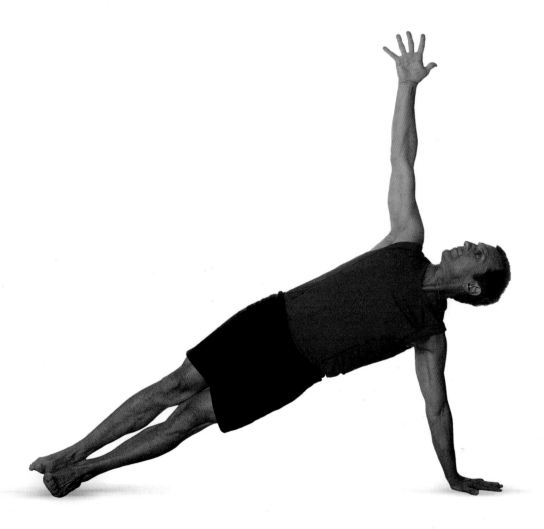

Plank, Side Extended

Utthita Vasisthasana

Difficulty Level   7

Start Position   Plank, side (p. 107)

1 Curl first two fingers around left (top) big toe.

2 Extend left leg upward. Repeat on other side.

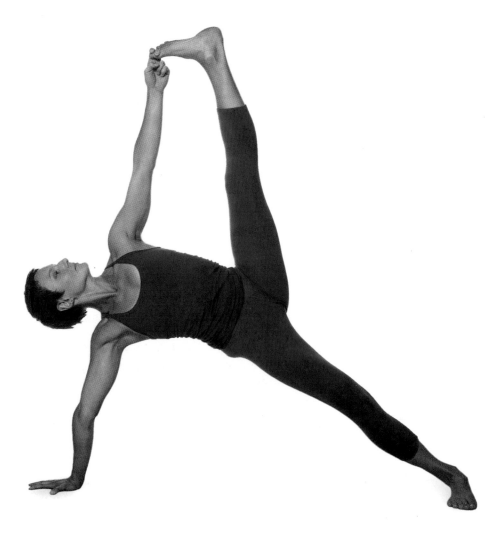

Plow

Halasana

Difficulty Level   4

Start Position   **Reclining on back**

1 Lift feet up and overhead until toes touch floor behind head.

2 Straighten arms and interlace fingers behind back.

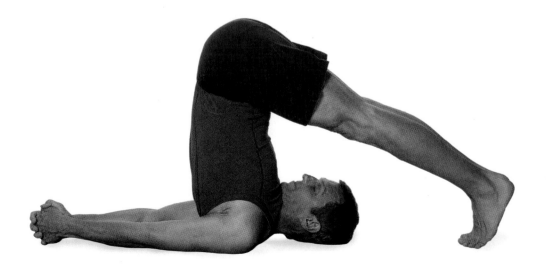

Plow, Side

Parsva Halasana

Difficulty Level   4

Start Position   Plow (p. 109)

1 Place hands on lower back.

2 Walk feet to left over left shoulder. Repeat on other side.

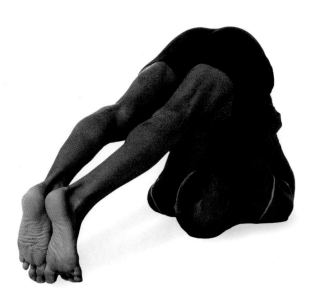

Pyramid

Parsvottanasana

Difficulty Level   4

Start Position   **Mountain, standing (p. 96)**

1 Step right foot forward so hips are square and outer left foot is grounded on floor.

2 Bend at hips and fold over right leg. Repeat on other side.

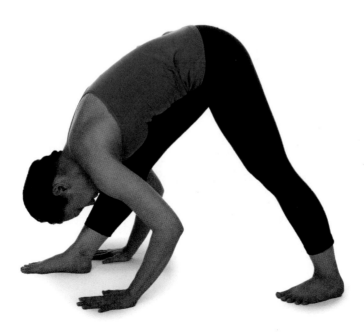

Reclining Angle

Supta Konasana

Difficulty Level   4

Start Position   Plow (p. 109)

1 Separate feet wide on floor overhead.

2 Curl first two fingers around big toes.

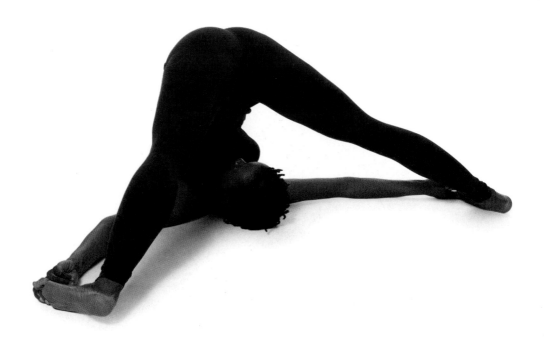

Sage

Siddhasana

Difficulty Level 1

Start Position Staff (p. 139)

1 Bend right knee.

2 Cross left ankle over right ankle.

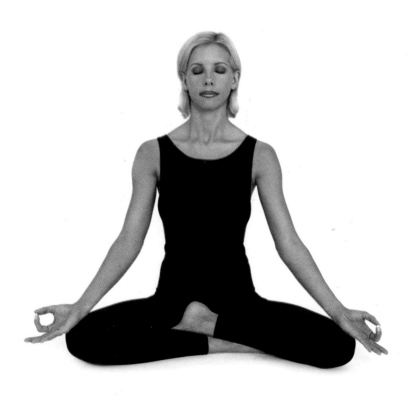

Sage Durva

Durvasana

Difficulty Level 9

Start Position Easy sitting (p. 41)

1 Hold outer right foot with left hand and duck head in front of right knee.

2 Place hands next to hips and press hips off floor.

3 Extend left leg straight up. Repeat on other side.

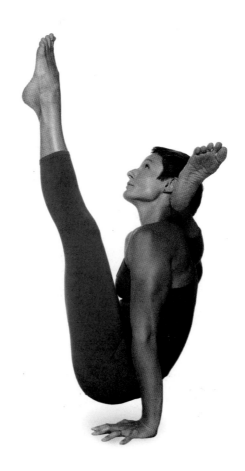

Sage Galava

Galavasana

Difficulty Level   5

Start Position   Mountain, standing (p. 96)

1 Bend left foot above right knee.

2 Sit down on right heel and balance with hands in prayer position. Repeat on other side.

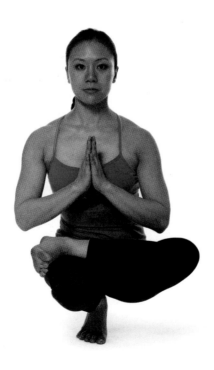

Sage Galava, One Leg

Eka Pada Galavasana

Difficulty Level 8

Start Position Sage Galava (p. 115)

1 Lean forward and place hands on floor.

2 Hook left shin on triceps with left foot flexed and lean forward, extending right leg back.

3 Balance on arms with chest and right leg parallel to floor. Repeat on other side.

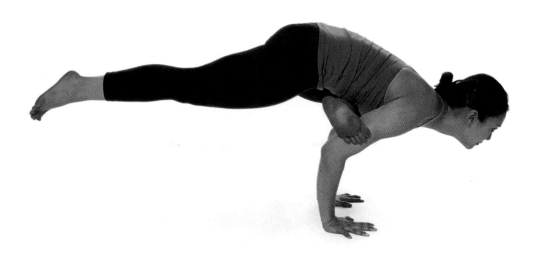

Sage Galava, Side One Leg

Parsva Eka Pada Galavasana

Difficulty Level   8

Start Position   Sage Galava (p. 115)

1 Rotate to left and hook left triceps under left foot.

2 Lean forward and place hands on floor, extending right leg straight out to side.

3 Balance on arms with chest and right leg parallel to floor. Repeat on other side.

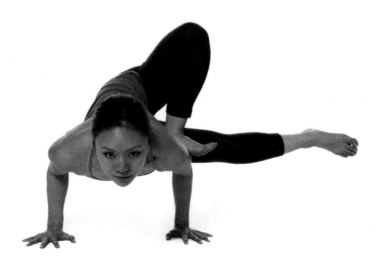

Sage Gheranda

Gherandasana

Difficulty Level 9

Start Position Locust (p. 85)

1 Bend right knee under left hip.

2 Reach right arm behind back and hold right foot.

3 Reach left arm overhead to catch left toes.

4 Kick left foot back for backbend. Repeat on other side.

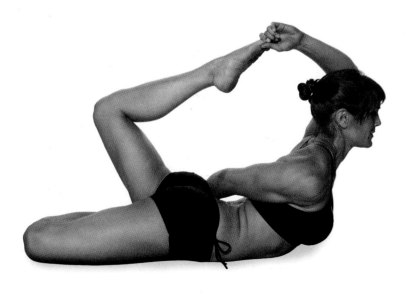

Sage Kasyapa

Kasyapasana

Difficulty Level   8

Start Position   **Plank, side (p. 107)**

1 Bend right (top) foot into left hip.

2 Reach right arm behind back to hold right foot.

3 Ground left inner foot. Repeat on other side.

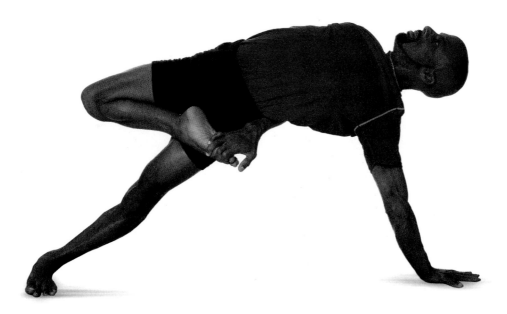

Sage Koundinya, One Leg

Eka Pada Koundinyasana I

Difficulty Level   7

Start Position   Crescent lunge (p. 31)

1 Place hands on floor to inside of left foot.

2 Hook left shoulder under left knee.

3 Balance on hands, extending left leg out and right leg straight back. Repeat on other side.

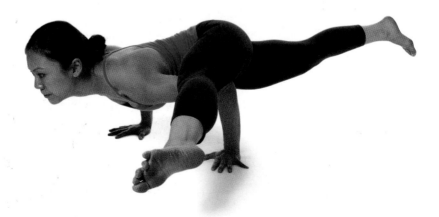

Sage Koundinya, Revolved One Leg

Eka Pada Koundinyasana II

Difficulty Level   8

Start Position   Crow, side (p. 35)

1 Separate legs by extending top leg back in the air and bottom leg straight out to side. Repeat on other side.

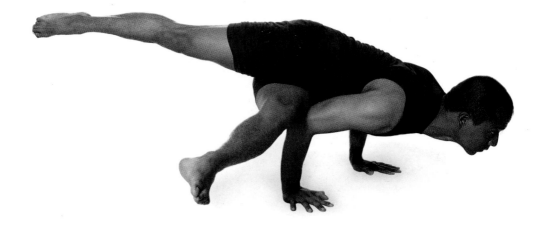

Sage Koundinya, Two Leg

Dwi Pada Koundinyasana

Difficulty Level 7

Start Position Crow, side (p. 35)

1 Extend both legs straight out to side. Repeat on other side.

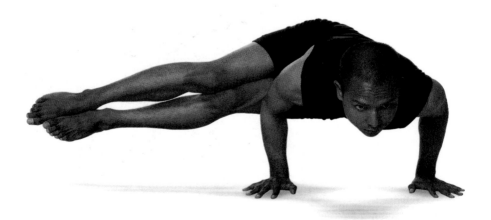

Sage Vamadeva

Vamadevasana

Difficulty Level 9

Start Position Pigeon, one-leg king of (p. 105)

1 Bend right (back) leg and hold right foot with right hand.

2 Twist torso to right and hold left foot toward right foot.

3 Gaze over right shoulder. Repeat on other side.

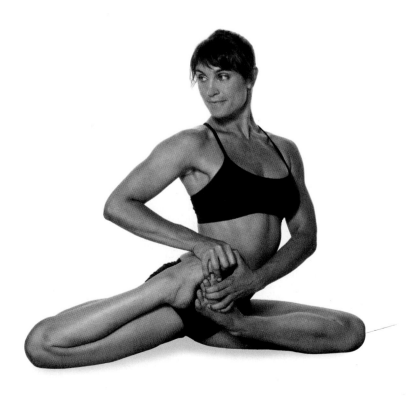

Sage Visvamitra

Visvamitrasana

Difficulty Level 9

Start Position Side angle, extended (p. 131)

1 Place right hand inside right foot and hook right shoulder under right knee.

2 Extend right leg off mat and straighten it forward, pressing right triceps into thigh for balance.

3 Extend left arm up. Repeat on other side.

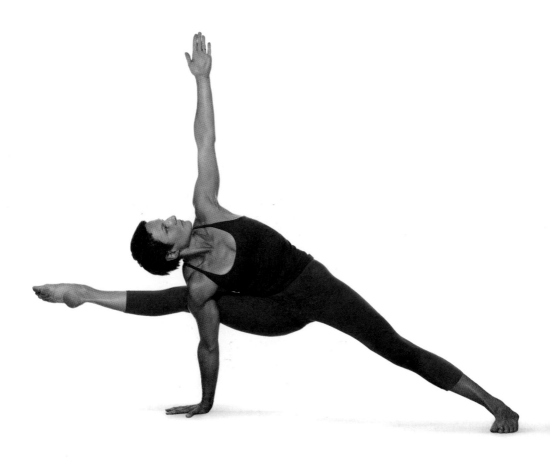

Scale

Tolasana

Difficulty Level 8

Start Position Lotus, seated (p. 90)

1 Place hands next to hips.

2 Press into hands to lift hips and balance, keeping legs in lotus.

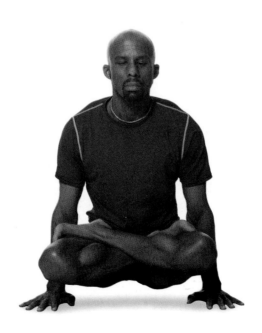

Scorpion I

Vrschikasana I

Difficulty Level   8

Start Position   Peacock feathers (forearm stand) (p. 101)

1 Bend knees and point toes to head.

2 Extend chest forward and up.

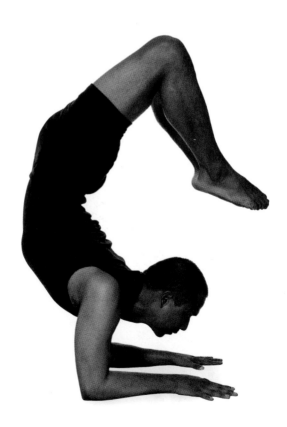

Scorpion II

Vrschikasana II

Difficulty Level 10

Start Position Handstand (p. 67)

1 Bend knees and point toes to head.

2 Extend chest forward and up.

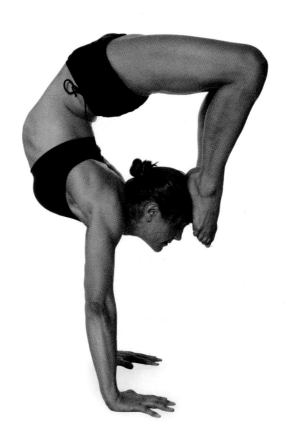

Shoulder Press

Bhujapidasana

Difficulty Level   8

Start Position   Garland I (p. 60)

1 Lift hips and walk hands back under buttocks.

2 Rest knees over shoulders.

3 Lift feet off floor. Cross ankles and straighten arms.

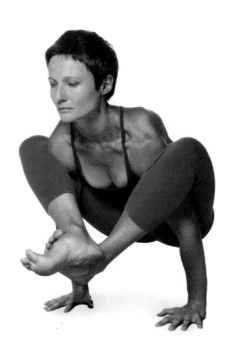

Shoulder Stand, Side Twist

Parsva Sarvangasana

Difficulty Level   6

Start Position   Plow (p. 109)

1 Place right hand behind sacrum.

2 Rotate hips to right.

3 Extend legs toward floor. Repeat on other side.

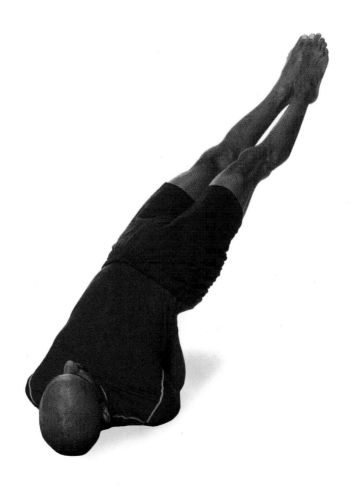

Shoulder Stand, Supported

Salamba Sarvangasana

Difficulty Level 5

Start Position Plow (p. 109)

1 Place hands on lower back.

2 Extend legs straight upward.

3 Press hips over shoulders.

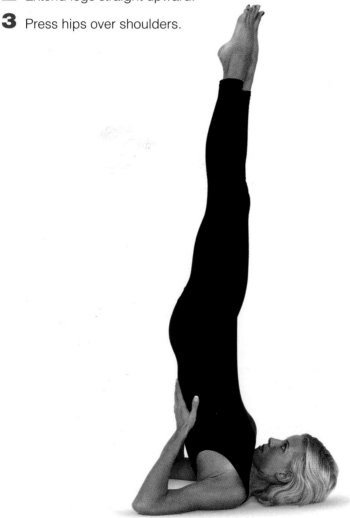

Side Angle, Extended

Utthita Parsvakonasana

Difficulty Level   4

Start Position   Warrior II (p. 152)

1 Place left hand on floor outside left (front) foot.

2 Extend right arm up or overhead and stack hips. Repeat on other side.

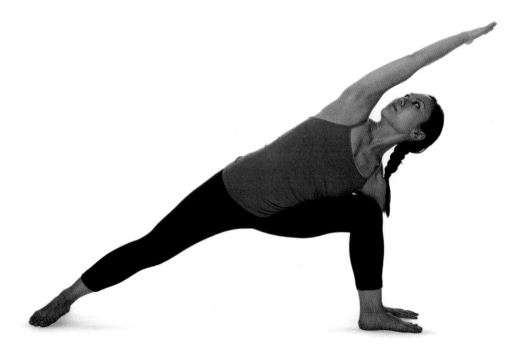

Side Angle, Revolved

Parivrtta Parsvakonasana

Difficulty Level 5

Start Position Side angle, extended (p. 131)

1 Rotate torso and place right hand on floor outside left foot.

2 Extend left arm up or overhead. Repeat on other side.

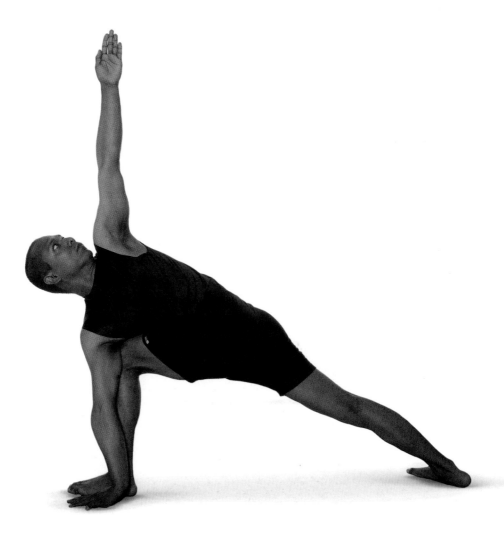

Son of Brahma I

Marichyasana I

Difficulty Level   5

Start Position   Staff (p. 139)

1 Bend right knee, placing foot on floor.

2 Extend right arm inside right bent leg, and wrap arm around leg.

3 Clasp left wrist with right hand behind back and fold over left straight leg. Repeat on other side.

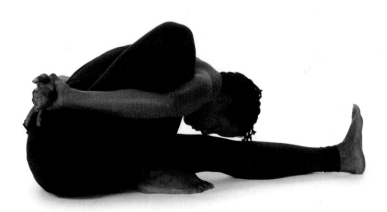

Son of Brahma II

Marichyasana II

Difficulty Level 7

Start Position Staff (p. 139)

1 Bend right knee, rotating right foot into left hip.

2 Bend left knee, placing left foot on floor and keeping right foot in hip crease.

3 Extend left arm under left leg and bind hands behind back. Repeat on other side.

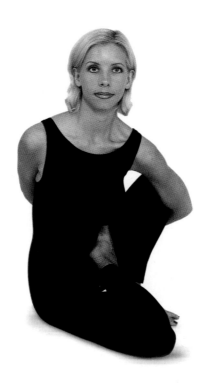

Son of Brahma III

Marichyasana III

Difficulty Level   6

Start Position   Staff (p. 139)

1 Bend left knee, placing foot on floor.

2 Rotate torso to left and hook right elbow on outside of left leg.

3 Place left hand on floor behind back or bind hands. Repeat on other side.

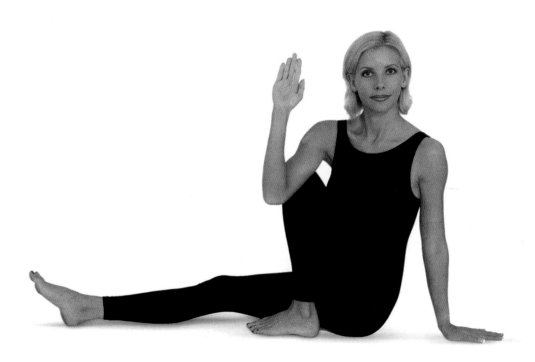

Sphinx

Difficulty Level 3

Start Position Lying on belly

1 Press up onto forearms with elbows under shoulders.

2 Lift chest and relax shoulders.

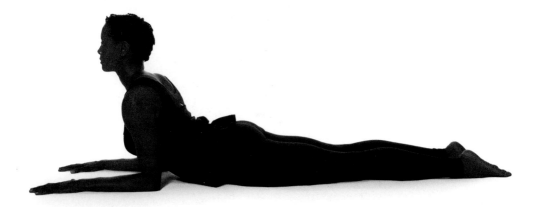

Spinal Twist

Jathara Parivartanasana

Difficulty Level 4

Start Position Reclining on back

1 Extend legs upward and to right until bottom leg rests on floor.

2 Open arms out to sides. Repeat on other side.

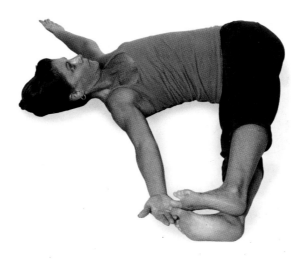

Splits, Forward

Hanumanasana

Difficulty Level 6

Start Position Crescent lunge (p. 31)

1 Slide right leg forward until thighs rest on floor.

2 Internally rotate back leg. Repeat on other side.

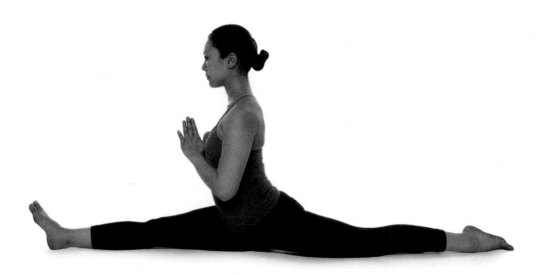

Staff

Dandasana

Difficulty Level   2

Start Position   Seated

1 Sit upright and extend legs forward.

2 Flex feet and engage abdomen.

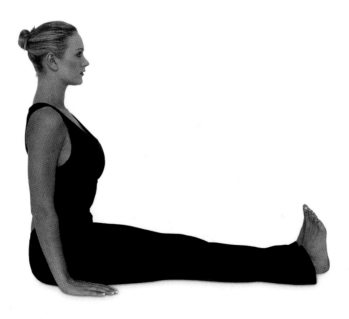

Staff, Four Limb

Chaturanga Dandasana

Difficulty Level   5

Start Position   Plank (p. 106)

1 Gazing slightly forward, bend elbows to shoulder height alongside body.

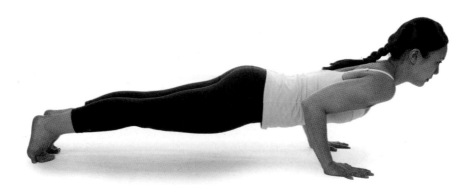

Straight Angle

Samakonasana

Difficulty Level   6

Start Position   Staff (p. 139)

1 Extend one leg at a time to sides.

2 Shift buttocks forward so that feet are parallel with hips.

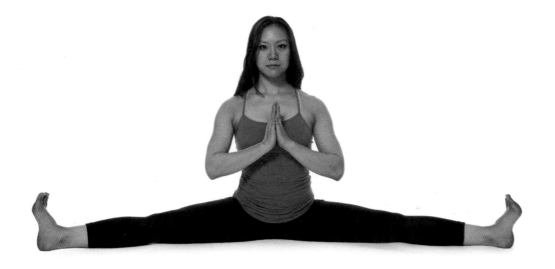

Three Steps, Reclining

Supta Trivkramasana

Difficulty Level 5

Start Position **Reclining on back**

1 Extend right leg up next to head.

2 Hold right foot with both hands. Repeat on other side.

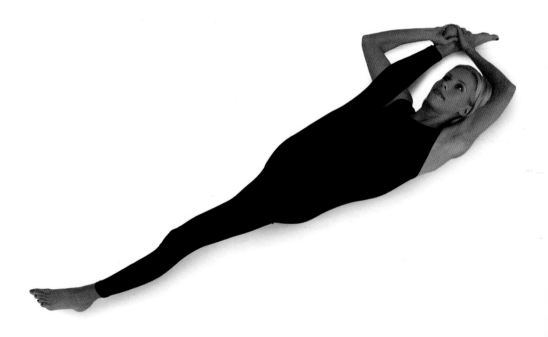

Tortoise

Kurmasana

Difficulty Level 5

Start Position Garland I (p. 60)

1 Bring sit bones to floor, keeping knees bent.

2 Reach arms under knees and straighten legs until chest meets floor.

3 Extend arms out to sides.

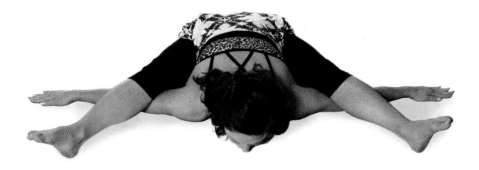

Tortoise, Bound

Baddha Kurmasana

Difficulty Level   7

Start Position   Garland I (p. 60)

1 Bring sit bones to floor, keeping knees bent.

2 Reach arms under knees and straighten legs until chest meets floor.

3 Bind hands behind back.

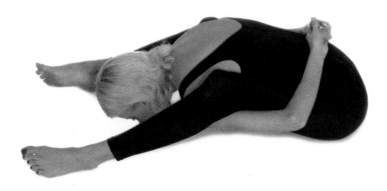

Tree

Vrksasana

Difficulty Level   4

Start Position   Mountain, standing (p. 96)

1 Step right foot onto inner left leg.

2 Extend arms upward. Repeat on other side.

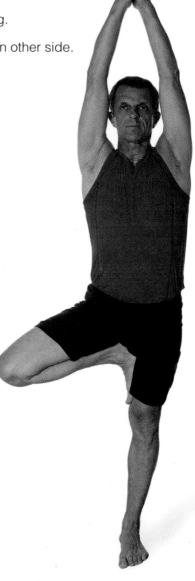

Triangle, Extended

Utthita Trikonasana

Difficulty Level 4

Start Position Warrior II (p. 152)

1 Straighten right (front) leg and extend torso forward.

2 Extend left arm up and right arm to floor. Repeat on other side.

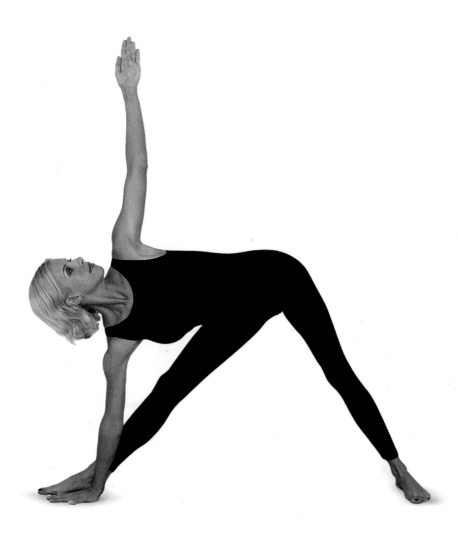

Triangle, Revolved

Parivrtta Trikonasana

Difficulty Level 5

Start Position Warrior II (p. 152)

1 Straighten right (front) leg and square torso forward.

2 Place left hand on outside of right foot.

3 Extend right hand straight up. Repeat on other side.

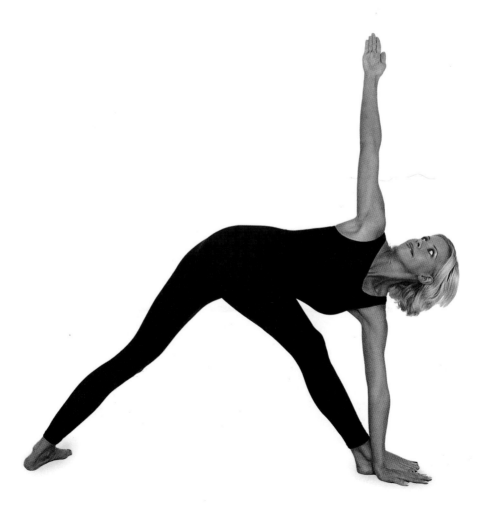

Upward-Facing Dog

Urdhva Mukha Svanasana

Difficulty Level 4

Start Position Cobra (p. 20)

1 Press into hands, straighten arms, and lift knees and thighs off floor.

2 Open chest, relax shoulders, and press into tops of feet.

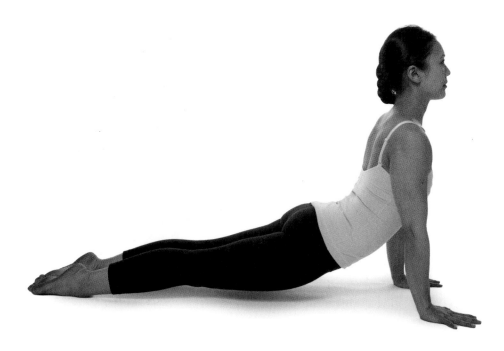

Upward-Facing Intense Stretch

Tiriang Mukhottanasana

Difficulty Level   10

Start Position   Mountain, standing (p. 96)

1 Lean back and press hips forward, bracing hands on lower back.

2 Reach arms overhead and walk hands down legs until hands clasp ankles.

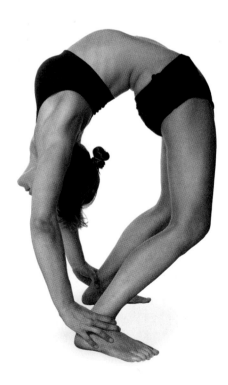

Upward-Facing Leg Stretch

Uttana Padasana

Difficulty Level   4

Start Position   Fish (p. 46)

1 Extend legs up to 45-degree angle, keeping crown of head on floor.

2 Reach arms up parallel to legs and connect hands.

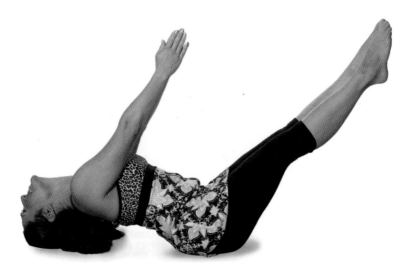

Warrior I

Virabhadrasana I

Difficulty Level   4

Start Position   Mountain, standing (p. 96)

1 Step right leg forward and bend knee.

2 Pivot left foot to a 45-degree angle.

3 Square hips to front and reach arms overhead. Repeat on other side.

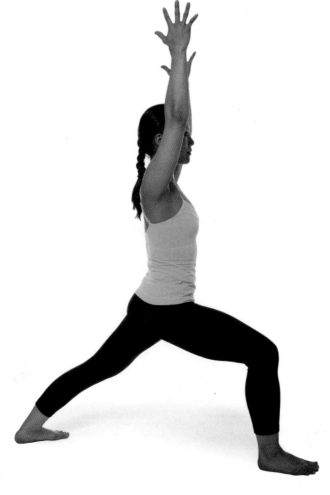

Warrior II

Virabhadrasana II

Difficulty Level 4

Start Position Mountain, standing (p. 96)

1 Step left leg forward and bend knee.

2 Pivot right foot to a 90-degree angle.

3 Square hips to side and reach arms to both sides. Repeat on other side.

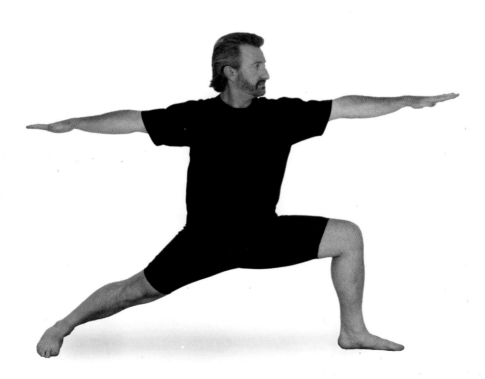

Warrior III

Virabhadrasana III

Difficulty Level 5

Start Position Mountain, standing (p. 96)

1 Extend left leg back in the air with foot flexed and toes pointing down.

2 Extend arms overhead, keeping both legs straight.

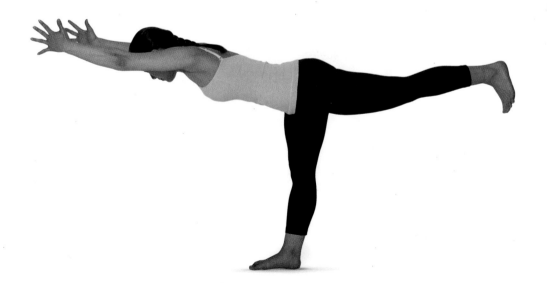

Wheel, Full

Urdhva Dhanurasana

Difficulty Level   5

Start Position   **Reclining on back**

1 Bend knees, placing feet on floor.

2 Place hands alongside head.

3 Press up, straightening arms.

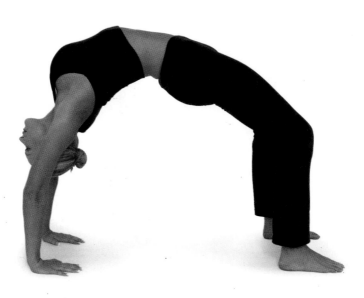

Wheel, One Leg Upward

Eka Pada Urdhva Dhanurasana

Difficulty Level 6

Start Position Wheel, full (p. 154)

1 Extend left leg straight up. Repeat on other side.

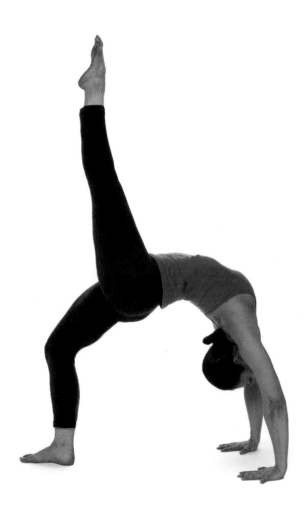

Wind Relieving

Pavanamuktasana

Difficulty Level   1

Start Position   **Reclining on back**

1 Bend both knees into chest and hug arms around legs.

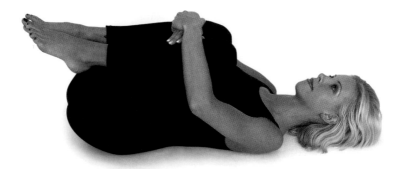

Yoga Mudra

Yoga Mudrasana

Difficulty Level   6

Start Position   Lotus, seated bound (p. 91)

1 Fold forward, keeping hands on feet.

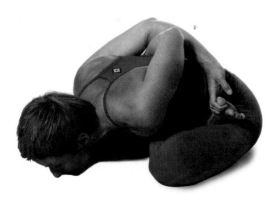

Yogic Sleep

Yoganidrasana

Difficulty Level 8

Start Position **Reclining on back**

1 Lift head to hook left foot behind head.

2 Hook right foot over left foot behind head and bind hands behind back.

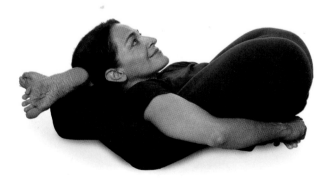

Sun Salutation

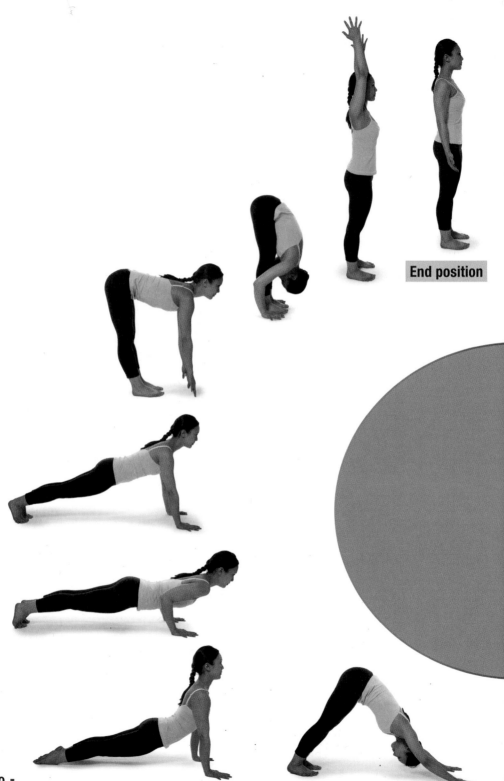

End position

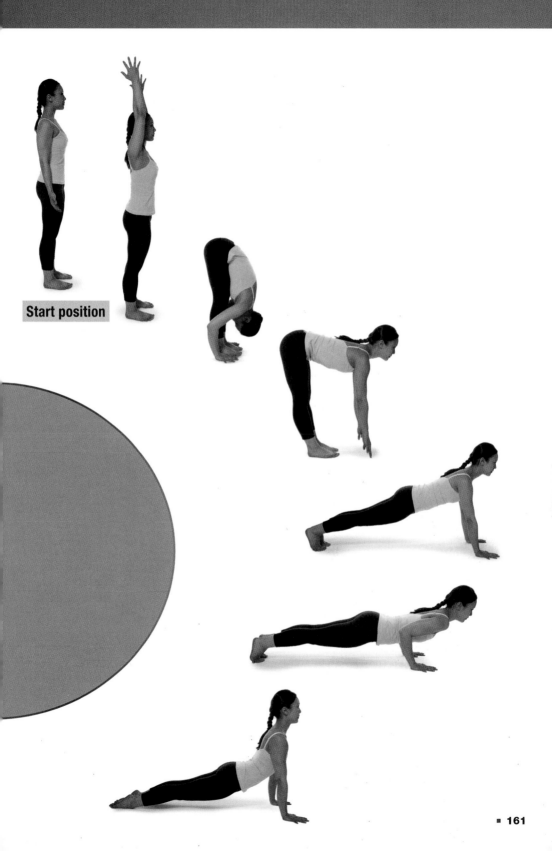

Start position

Suggested Readings

Chodron, Pema. 2001. *The wisdom of no escape and the path of loving kindness.* Boston: Shambhala.

Desikachar, T.K.V. 1995. *The heart of yoga.* Rochester, NY: Inner Traditions.

Gannon, Sharon, and David Life. 2002. *Jivamukti yoga.* New York: Ballantine Books.

Iyengar, B.K.S. 1977. *Light on yoga: Yoga dipika.* New York: Schocken Books.

Kirk, Martin, Brooke Boon, and Daniel DiTuro. 2005. *Hatha yoga illustrated.* Illinois: Human Kinetics.

Lasater, P.T., and Judith Hanson. 2009. *Yoga body: Anatomy, kinesiology and asana.* Berkeley, CA: Rodmell Press.

Lee, Cyndi. 2004. *Yoga body, Buddha mind.* New York: Riverhead Books.

Long, Ray, and Chris Macivor. 2006. *The key muscles of yoga: Scientific keys, Volume I.* (3rd ed.). Baldwinsville, NY: BandhaYoga.

McCall, Timothy. 2007. *Yoga as medicine: The yogic prescription for health and healing.* New York: Bantam Books.

Mehta, Silva, Mira Mehta, and Shyam Mehta. 2003. *Yoga: The Iyengar way.* New York: Knopf.

Miller, Richard. 2010. *Yoga nidra: A meditative practice for deep relaxation and healing.* Lousville, CO: Sounds True.

Rountree, Sage. 2008. *The athlete's guide to yoga.* Boulder, CO: Velopress.

Satchidananda, Sri Swami. 1978. *The yoga sutras of Patanjali.* Yogaville, VA: Integral Yoga.

Swenson, David. 1999. *Ashtanga yoga: The practice manual.* Texas: Ashtanga Yoga.

Resources

Resource for detailed descriptions of yoga poses:

www.yogajournal.com

Resource for yoga props, equipment and accessories:

www.yogaaccessories.com

The authors are grateful for the use of Prana Yoga Center and Yoga Is Youthfulness for photographing many of the asanas appearing in this book.

Prana Yoga Center
1041 Silverado St.
La Jolla, CA 92037
858-456-2806
E-mail: info@prana-yoga.com
Website: www.prana-yoga.com

Yoga Is Youthfulness
590 Castro Street
Mountain View, CA 94041
650-964-5277
E-mail: info@yogaisyouth.com
Website: www.yogaisyouth.com

Index of Asanas

English Names in Alphabetical Order

Sanskrit Names in Alphabetical Order

* No Sanskrit equivalent exists for this English term.

About the Authors

A self-taught photographer, **Daniel DiTuro** began a series of yoga photographs in 1999 shortly after taking his first yoga class. In 2001 he began The Yoga Project to promote the physical and mental wellness of mind, body, and spirit through the creation and publication of inspirational and motivational meditation and yoga asana photographs. In 2003, DiTuro, along with Martin Kirk and Brooke Boone, released the best-seller *Hatha Yoga Illustrated*, which contains over 600 of his yoga photographs.

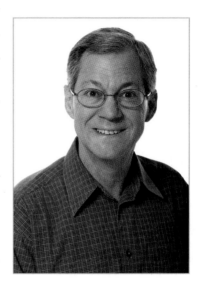

DiTuro published his second book, *Live Longer & Healthier Eating Foods You Love on a Southern Italian Mediterranean Diet*, in August 2009, which was one of the selections for the United States in the 2010 Gourmand World Cookbook Awards.

Coauthor **Ingrid Yang** embarked on her yoga journey in 1999 in New York City, where she studied directly with David Life at Jivamukti Yoga Center and Cyndi Lee at OM Yoga Center. She is the founder of Blue Point Yoga Center in Durham, North Carolina, and teaches a variety of yoga disciplines, including vinyasa, restorative, yin, and cancer therapy. She leads teacher trainings and workshops in the United States, Australia, and Asia.

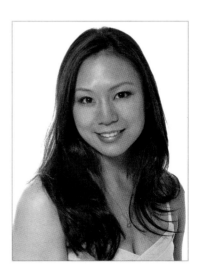

Ingrid earned her law degree at Duke University and is currently pursuing a doctor of medicine degree with a focus on anatomy and physiatry at Rush University Medical College in Chicago, Illinois.

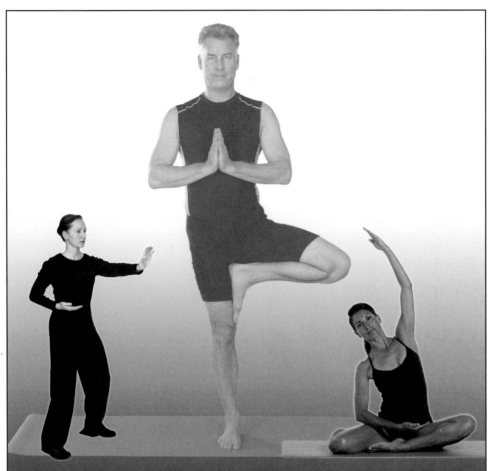